Peripheral Nerve Conditions: Using Evidence to Guide Treatment

Editor

WARREN C. HAMMERT

HAND CLINICS

www.hand.theclinics.com

Consulting Editor
KEVIN C. CHUNG

August 2013 • Volume 29 • Number 3

ELSEVIER

1600 John F. Kennedy Boulevard • Suite 1800 • Philadelphia, Pennsylvania, 19103-2899

http://www.theclinics.com

HAND CLINICS Volume 29, Number 3
August 2013 ISSN 0749-0712, ISBN-13: 978-0-323-24199-1

Editor: Jennifer Flynn-Briggs

Hand Clinics (ISSN 0749-0712) is published quarterly by Elsevier Inc., 360 Park Avenue South, New York, NY 10010-1710. Months of publication are February, May, August, and November. Business and Editorial Offices: 1600 John F. Kennedy Blvd., Ste. 1800, Philadelphia, PA 19103-2899. Customer Service Office: 3251 Riverport Lane, Maryland Heights, MO 63043. Periodicals postage paid at New York, NY and at additional mailing offices. Subscription price is $390.00 per year (domestic individuals), $606.00 per year (domestic institutions), $194.00 per year (domestic students/residents), $445.00 per year (Canadian individuals), $691.00 per year (Canadian institutions), $530.00 per year (international individuals), $691.00 per year (international institutions), and $256.00 per year (international and Canadian students/residents). Foreign air speed delivery is included in all *Clinics* subscription prices. All prices are subject to change without notice. **POSTMASTER:** Send address changes to *Hand Clinics*, Elsevier Health Sciences Division, Subscription Customer Service, 3251 Riverport Lane, Maryland Heights, MO 63043. Customer Service (orders, claims, online, change of address): Elsevier Health Sciences Division, Subscription Customer Service, 3251 Riverport Lane, Maryland Heights, MO 63043. Tel: 1-800-654-2452 (U.S. and Canada); 314-447-8871 (outside U.S. and Canada). Fax: 314-447-8029. E-mail: journalscustomerservice-usa@elsevier.com (for print support); journalsonlinesupport-usa@elsevier.com (for online support).

Reprints. For copies of 100 or more of articles in this publication, please contact the Commercial Reprints Department, Elsevier Inc., 360 Park Avenue South, New York, New York 10010-1710. Tel.: 212-633-3812; Fax: 212-462-1935; E-mail: reprints@elsevier.com.

Hand Clinics is covered in *MEDLINE/PubMed (Index Medicus), Current Contents/Clinical Medicine, EMBASE/Excerpta Medica,* and *ISI/BIOMED.*

Printed and bound by CPI Group (UK) Ltd, Croydon, CR0 4YY

Transferred to digital print 2012

Contributors

CONSULTING EDITOR

KEVIN C. CHUNG, MD, MS
Charles B.G. de Nancrede Professor of
Surgery, Section of Plastic Surgery,
Department of Surgery, Assistant Dean for
Faculty Affairs, Associate Director of Global
REACH, University of Michigan Medical
School, University of Michigan Health System,
Ann Arbor, Michigan

EDITOR

WARREN C. HAMMERT, MD
Associate Professor of Orthopaedics and
Plastic Surgery, Department of Orthopaedic
Surgery, University of Rochester Medical
Center, Rochester, New York

AUTHORS

ERIK R. BERGQUIST, MD
Fellow, Hand and Upper Extremity Fellowship,
Department of Orthopaedic Surgery, University
of Rochester Medical Center, Rochester,
New York

DAVID M. BROGAN, MD, MSc
Resident Physician, Department of Orthopedic
Surgery, Mayo Clinic, Rochester, Minnesota

RYAN P. CALFEE, MD, MSc
Assistant Professor, Department of
Orthopaedic Surgery, Washington University
School of Medicine, Washington University,
St Louis, Missouri

IAN CARROLL, MD, MS
Assistant Professor, Department of
Anesthesia, Stanford University, Palo Alto,
California

PETER C. CHIMENTI, MD
Resident, Department of Orthopaedics,
University of Rochester Medical Center,
Rochester, New York

KEVIN C. CHUNG, MD, MS
Charles B.G. de Nancrede Professor
of Surgery, Section of Plastic Surgery,
Department of Surgery, Assistant Dean
for Faculty Affairs, Associate Director of
Global REACH, University of Michigan
Medical School, University of Michigan
Health System, Ann Arbor, Michigan

CATHERINE M. CURTIN, MD
Staff Physician, Palo Alto VA; Assistant
Professor, Division of Plastic Surgery,
Stanford University, Palo Alto,
California

JOHN C. ELFAR, MD
Department of Orthopaedics, University
of Rochester Medical Center, Rochester,
New York

THERON S. FUSSELL, BA
School of Medicine and Dentistry, University
of Rochester Medical Center, Rochester,
New York

RANJAN GUPTA, MD
Professor & Chair, Department of Orthopaedic
Surgery, University of California Irvine, Irvine,
California

WARREN C. HAMMERT, MD
Associate Professor of Orthopaedic and
Plastic Surgery, Department of Orthopaedic
Surgery, University of Rochester Medical
Center, Rochester, New York

THOMAS B. HUGHES, MD
Associate Professor of Orthopaedic Surgery,
University of Pittsburgh School of Medicine,
UPMC, Pittsburgh, Pennsylvania

JONATHAN ISAACS, MD
Chair, Division of Hand Surgery, Department of
Orthopaedic Surgery, Virginia Commonwealth
University Health System, Richmond, Virginia

SANJEEV KAKAR, MD, MRCS
Associate Professor of Orthopedics,
Department of Orthopedic Surgery, Mayo
Clinic, Rochester, Minnesota

ELISA J. KNUTSEN, MD
Fellow, Department of Orthopaedic Surgery,
Washington University School of Medicine,
Washington University, St Louis, Missouri

MICHAEL Y. LIN, MD, PhD
Orthopaedic Surgery Resident PGY5,
Department of Orthopaedic Surgery, University
of California Irvine, Irvine, California

GIVENCHY MANZANO, BS
Medical Student Year 3, Department of
Orthopaedic Surgery, University of California
Irvine, Irvine, California

CLIFTON G. MEALS, MD
Department of Orthopedics, George
Washington University Medical Center,
Washington, DC

ROY A. MEALS, MD
Department of Orthopedics, University
of California Los Angeles Medical Center,
Los Angeles, California

RON M.G. MENORCA, BS
School of Medicine and Dentistry, University
of Rochester Medical Center, Rochester,
New York

BRIAN A. MOSIER, MD
Resident, Department of Orthopaedics,
Allegheny General Hospital, Pittsburgh,
Pennsylvania

CHRISTINE B. NOVAK, PT, PhD
Associate Professor, Department of Surgery,
University of Toronto; Scientist, Toronto
Rehab, University Health Network; Research
Associate, Hand Program, University Health
Network, Toronto, Ontario, Canada

DAVID RING, MD, PhD
Chief, MGH Hand Service, Massachusetts
General Hospital; Associate Professor of
Orthopaedic Surgery, Harvard Medical School,
Boston, Massachusetts

MALAY SUNITHA, MPH
Clinical Research Coordinator, Section of
Plastic Surgery, Department of Surgery,
University of Michigan Health System,
Ann Arbor, Michigan

**REBECCA L. VON DER HEYDE, PhD, OTR/L,
CHT**
Associate Professor, Director of the
Occupational Therapy Department, Concordia
University Wisconsin, Mequon, Wisconsin

YIRONG WANG, MD
Plastic Surgery Hospital, Peking Union Medical
College, Chinese Academy of Medical
Science, Beijing, China

Contents

other noxious stimuli over the regenerating nerve end. The choice of treatment depends in part on the nerve affected, whether it involves critical or noncritical sensation, and its location.

HAND CLINICS

Preface

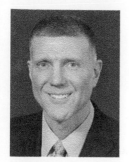

Warren C. Hammert, MD
Editor

Injuries and other conditions affecting the peripheral nervous system present a challenge for the hand and upper extremity surgeon and, in some cases, are life altering for the patient.

Ideally, every nerve injury would follow a predictable sequence, resulting in a perfect recovery and every compressive neuropathy would have a straightforward treatment with predictable outcomes. Unfortunately, this is often not the case and the surgeon must have a plan for management of these conditions. Evidence-based medicine should guide our treatment to minimize complications and provide the most optimal outcomes for our patients. For many conditions involving the upper extremity peripheral nervous system, evidence is scarce and we must rely on studies involving level III and level IV evidence.

My goal in organizing this edition of *Hand Clinics* was to provide the reader with a review of many challenging upper extremity peripheral nerve topics, which are rarely grouped together, providing an evidence-based approach to their management, focusing on outcomes. I think you will find this is different than what you will find in the traditional hand surgery textbooks.

I would like to thank all of the esteemed contributors for their time and efforts, without which, this edition would not have been possible. In addition, a special thanks to Jennifer Flynn-Briggs, Yonah Korngold, David Parsons, and Elsevier for their professional assistance from the idea, through the development, and ultimately, publication of this issue of *Hand Clinics*.

Warren C. Hammert, MD
Department of Orthopaedic Surgery
University of Rochester Medical Center
601 Elmwood Avenue, Box 665
Rochester, NY 14642, USA

E-mail address:
Warren_Hammert@URMC.Rochester.edu

Hand Clin 29 (2013) ix
http://dx.doi.org/10.1016/j.hcl.2013.04.015

Nerve Physiology
Mechanisms of Injury and Recovery

Ron M.G. Menorca, BS[a], Theron S. Fussell, BA[a],
John C. Elfar, MD[b],*

KEYWORDS

- Nerve physiology • Nerve injury • Nerve recovery • Peripheral nerve injuries

KEY POINTS

- Peripheral nerve injuries are common and can be debilitating, leading to poor quality of life. Available treatments remain suboptimal. Injuries range in severity from mild compression to severe crush and lacerations.
- Classification schemes describing the extent of injury provide clinicians and scientists with a language to correlate nerve pathophysiology with patient symptoms and prognosis.
- In vivo injury models, in particular the sciatic nerve of rodents, have been used extensively to study the effectiveness of both surgical and medical treatments for nerve injury, using appropriate outcome measurements.
- Experiments using cell cultures have elucidated interactions among nerve cell constituents and revealed the complex interplay between factors in the injury microenvironment.
- Taken together, advancements in the understanding of nerve injury and recovery continue to provide new avenues for surgeons to explore future prospective therapies.

INTRODUCTION

Peripheral nerve injuries are common conditions with broad-ranging groups of symptoms, depending on the severity and nerves involved. Although much knowledge exists on the mechanisms of injury and regeneration, reliable treatments that ensure full functional recovery are scarce. This review aims to summarize various ways these injuries are classified in light of decades of research on peripheral nerve injury and regeneration.

PERIPHERAL NERVE ANATOMY

The peripheral nervous system comprises 3 types of cells: neuronal cells, glial cells, and stromal cells. Peripheral nerves convey signals between the spinal cord and the rest of the body. Nerves are composed of various combinations of motor, sensory, and autonomic neurons. Efferent neurons (motor and autonomic) receive signals through their dendrites from neurons of the central nervous system, primarily using the neurotransmitter acetylcholine. Afferent (sensory) neurons receive their signals through their dendrites from specialized cell types, such as pacinian corpuscles for fine sensation. These signals are sent to the central nervous system to provide sensory information to the brain and possibly interneurons in the spinal cord when a reflex response is necessary.[1]

Key roles are played by cells other than neurons in the maintenance and function of the peripheral nerves. Schwann cells ensheath nerves in a layer of myelin and provide trophic support through the release of important neurotrophs, such as nerve growth factor (NGF). Myelin improves conduction velocity by limiting the sites of ionic

The authors of this article have nothing to disclose.
a School of Medicine and Dentistry, University of Rochester Medical Center, 601 Elmwood Avenue, Box 665, Rochester, NY 14642, USA; b Department of Orthopaedics, University of Rochester Medical Center, 601 Elmwood Avenue, Box 665, Rochester, NY 14642, USA
* Corresponding author.
E-mail address: openelfar@gmail.com

Hand Clin 29 (2013) 317–330
http://dx.doi.org/10.1016/j.hcl.2013.04.002
0749-0712/13/$ – see front matter © 2013 Published by Elsevier Inc

transfer along the axon to the nodes of Ranvier, resulting in a faster, jumping action potential propagation that is termed, *saltatory conduction*. The most heavily myelinated fibers are the large motor neurons (type Aα), followed by afferent muscle spindles (type Aβ). Nerve conduction velocities in theses neurons are approximately 30 m/s to 120 m/s. Unmyelinated neurons (type C), such as the sensory neurons involved in transmitting pain and temperature and postganglionic sympathetics, are the slowest, conducting at approximately 1 m/s to 2 m/s (**Table 1**).[2,3]

The non-neuronal cells and connective tissues surrounding neuronal axons provide a complex stromal connective tissue scaffold[4] for the nerve and are important in understanding and classifying nerve injuries. Encasing the individual axons is the deepest structural layer, the endoneurium. Surrounding the endoneurium, the perineurium circumferentially bundles axons together to form fascicles. The outermost connective tissue layer of the nerve, the epineurium, consists of 2 parts. Dispersed between fascicles is the epifascicular epineurium whereas surrounding the nerve trunk proper is the epineural epinerium. Microvessels progressively branch through the nerve according to the structural layers, providing blood to the axons. Due to their more peripheral location,

epineural vessels are more susceptible to trauma than the deeper vessels in the nerve.[5]

CLASSIFICATIONS OF NERVE INJURIES

Peripheral nerve injuries pose various challenges to patients, ranging from mild discomfort to lifelong impairment. A classification scheme provides a common language for physicians and scientists to effectively discuss nerve pathophysiology (**Table 2**). Seddon[6] was the first to classify nerve injuries into 3 categories based on the presence of demyelination and the extent of damage to the axons and the connective tissues of the nerve. The mildest form of injury is called neurapraxia, defined by focal demyelination without damage to the axons or the connective tissues. Neurapraxia typically occurs from mild compression or traction of the nerve and results in a decrease in conduction velocity. Depending on the severity of demyelination, the effects can range from asynchronous conduction to conduction block, causing muscle weakness. The next level is called axonotmesis, which involves direct damage to the axons in addition to focal demyelination while maintaining continuity of the nerve's connective tissues. The most severe form of injury is called neurotmesis, which is a full transection of the

Table 1
Nerve fiber types and properties

Fiber Class	Myelin	Diameter (μm)	Conduction Velocity (m/s)	Spinal Cord Tract	Location	Function
Aα	+	6–22	30–120	Ipsilateral dorsal column	Efferent to muscles	Motor
Aβ	+	6–22	30–120	Contralateral spinothalamic tract	Afferent from skin and joints	Tactile, proprioception
Aγ	+	3–8	15–35	Ipsilateral dorsal column	Efferent to muscle spindles	Muscle tone
Aδ	+	1–4	5–30	Contralateral spinothalamic tract	Afferent sensory nerves	Pain, cold, temperature, touch
B	+	1–3	3–15	Preganglionic	Preganglionic sympathetic	Various autonomic functions
sC	−	0.3–1.3	0.7–1.3	—	Postganglionic sympathetic	Various autonomic functions
dC	−	0.4–1.2	0.1–2.0	Contralateral spinothalamic tract	Afferent sensory nerves	Various autonomic functions Pain, warm, temperature, touch

Data from Berde CB, Strichartz GR. Local anesthetics. In: Miller R, Eriksson IL, Fleisher LA, et al, editors. Miller's anesthesia. 7th edition. Philadelphia: Elsevier, 2009; and Miner JR, Paris PM, Yealy DM. Pain management. In: Marx JA, Hockberger RS, Walls RM, et al, editors. Rosen's Emergency Medicine Concepts and Clinical Practice. Vol 2. 7th edition. Philadelphia: Saunders; 2010.

Table 2
Seddon and Sunderland classifications of nerve injury

Seddon	Sunderland	Injury
Neurapraxia	Grade I	Focal segmental demyelination
Axonotmesis	Grade II	Axon damaged with intact endoneurium
Axonotmesis	Grade III	Axon and endoneurium damaged with intact perineurium
Axonotmesis	Grade IV	Axon, endoneurium, and perineurium damaged with intact epineurium
Neurotmesis	Grade V	Complete nerve transection.
	Grade VI (MacKinnon and Dellon)	Mixed levels of injury along the nerve

axons and connective tissue layers, resulting in complete discontinuity of the nerve.

Sunderland[7] later expanded on this classification to distinguish the extent of damage in the connective tissues. In his classification scheme, grade I and grade V corresponded with Seddon's neurapraxia and neurotmesis, respectively. Grades II to IV, however, are all forms of axonotmesis, with increasing amounts of connective tissue damage. In grade II, axon damage is observed with no damage present in the connective tissue. Grade III involves damage to the endoneurium and grade IV includes damage to the perineurium (**Fig. 1**). A grade VI lesion was later introduced by Mackinnon and Dellon[8] to denote combinations of grades III to V injuries along a damaged nerve, although its usage has not been widely accepted. Attempts at simplifying this scheme by classifying nerves as either nondegenerative or degenerative were proposed by Thomas and Holdroff in 1993,[9] but the clinical significance of this simplification is still questionable.

COMPRESSION INJURY
Causes

Compression injuries are not always captured by the commonly used classification schemes. Nonetheless, there is little doubt that the majority of peripheral nerve compressions fall under the general class of neurapraxia, or grade I nerve injuries, and commonly occur in locations where nerves pass through narrow anatomic openings. The most common sites for compression injuries in the upper extremity are the carpal tunnel and the cubital tunnel. As is expected with a grade I nerve injury, compression injuries are defined by focal demyelination at the site of compression with the absence of axonal and connective tissue damage. Compressions can be acute or chronic in nature. Acute compressions, as seen in radial mononeuropathy, are commonly acquired after a night of external compression (ie, hanging one's arm over a chair) and typically present with transient paresthesia, numbness, and wrist drop. Complete recovery of the acutely compressed nerve can range from weeks to years. In contrast, chronic compressions, such as carpal tunnel syndrome, are progressively worsening conditions that persist without proper intervention. Symptoms may begin with paresthesia and distal numbness but, unlike acute compressions, often progress over time to muscle weakness and muscle wasting, depending on the extent of axonal damage at later stages.[10]

Pathophysiology

Light and electron microscopy demonstrate normal nerve morphology and neuromuscular junctions are present in chronic compression injuries.[11,12] A degraded, thinner myelin sheath is seen, however, as evidenced by an increased g ratio (ratio of the axon diameter to the axon plus myelin sheath diameter) and a decreased internodal length (distance between adjacent nodes of Ranvier). Other observations seen in the presence of this demyelination are Schwann cell proliferation, dedifferentiation, and an increase in Schmidt-Lanterman incisures, which are cytoplasmic components of Schwann cells that are thought to maintain the metabolism of the myelin sheath, so an increase in Schmidt-Lanterman incisures suggests that Schwann cells are increasing their metabolism to undergo remyelination in the presence of demyelination, as is typically seen in chronic compression injuries.[13]

There are various proposed mechanisms that are thought to lead to compression injuries.[14] From an anatomic standpoint, the narrowing of openings leads to increased pressure at that site, compressing blood vessels and leading to nerve ischemia, as occurs with vasculitis and artherosclerotic diseases. Another proposed mechanism

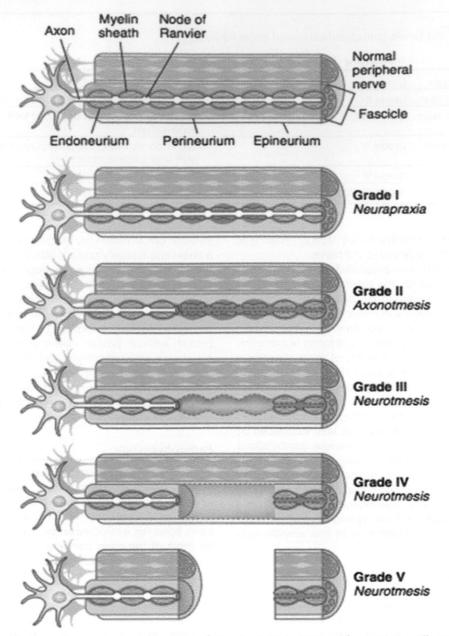

Fig. 1. Classification of nerve trauma. (*Courtesy of* Cleveland Clinic, 2006; with permission. Illustrator, David Schumick, BS, CMI.)

is the result of lower pressure, which decreases venous return and can lead to venous stasis. In this state, extraneural edema forms over time with subsequent fibrosis and scar tissue around the nerve and eventual intraneural edema. The examination of these 2 mechanisms begets the question of why the Schwann cells are chiefly affected and not the neurons themselves.

Chronic compression injury was once thought of as a milder form of wallerian degeneration. This

has long been disproved due to lack of axonal damage in this injury. The role of macrophages and their mitogenic factors, such as interleukin (IL) 1, IL-6, IL-10, and IL-12, in promoting Schwann cell activity has been proposed but is unlikely because Schwann cells are able to proliferate in the absence of macrophages.[15] Also, because the subtle gradual damage in chronic compression does not lead to an inflammatory response, macrophages arrive slowly and after much of the

Schwann cell proliferation has already occurred, further distancing macrophages from being the likely culprit.[16]

More recent studies have shown that shear stress alone can induce Schwann cell demyelination, proliferation, and remyelination.[17] These in vitro experiments were conducted in highly controlled chambers where gas concentrations, pressure, and solutes in the medium were regulated and monitored in real time. In such controlled conditions, the application of shear stresses leads to altered Schwann cell protein expression, with key changes attributed to altered expression of integrin β4.[17]

Much of the in vivo work for studying compression neuropathy has come from the use of biologically inert, polymeric silicone silastic tubes, more commonly used for surgical implants and prosthesis. These tubes have been used to create reliable models of compressive neuropathy in many animal models, such as rats,[18] rabbits,[19] and mice,[20] and have also been used to study double crush in vivo.[21] The compression neuropathy models are typically assessed by nerve conduction studies, which in these models reveal a gradual decline in nerve conduction velocities in the absence of neuronal or muscular damage, which would be evident if an altered compound muscle action potential was seen, but it was not.[14,19,23]

Double Crush

Within the realm of compression is another form of injury, known as double crush.[22] Double crush pertains to the increased susceptibility of a nerve to develop a compressive neuropathy when a proximal compressive lesion of the same nerve is found. This phenomenon was first defined by Upton and McComas in 1973[23] after an observation that 81 of 115 patients with carpal or cubital tunnel also had a neural lesion at the neck. The reverse form of double crush, aptly named reverse double crush, was later described by Dahlin and Lundborg in 1990,[24] after observing patients with an ulnar nerve entrapment at the wrist later developing a similar proximal injury at the elbow. The morphology of the lesion seen in double crush is identical to lesions seen in chronic compression, with the unique additive effect of multiple sites with otherwise subthreshold levels of pressure contributing to a suprathreshold effect on the nerve. The interruption of axonal traffic and flow may prove an explanation for how 2 minor areas of compression can collude to form an effect that mimics a greater compressive insult at a single site. An article by Wilbourn and Gilliatt in 1997[25]

discusses these models and their limitations and points out a need for further research and clinical overuse of the term, double crush, in cases that do not fit the specific parameters described by Upton and McComas and by Dahlin and Lundborg. The existence of double crush has been confirmed in various studies under subacute compression[26,27] and severe compression,[21] using animal nerves in vitro and in vivo.

CRUSH AND TRANSECTION INJURY
Causes

Crush injuries can cause many different degrees of neural damage that can represent any of the classes described by Seddon[6] or Sunderland.[7] Moreover, most of these injuries probably often represent mixed injuries of the sort suggested by Dellon and colleagues.[28,29]

Crush injuries typically occur from an acute traumatic compression of the nerve from a blunt object, such as a bat, surgical clamp, or other crushing object, that does not result in a complete transection of the nerve. In contrast, transection injuries, also known as neurotmesis or grade V nerve injuries, have a complete discontinuation of the nerve, commonly due to a laceration from a knife, gunshot, glass shard, and so forth.[30] Ballistic injuries are a special case that tends to combine both transection and crush of the nerve from the shockwave that moves through the tissue after the passage of the bullet, which has both a tearing and compressing effect on the nerve, even without the actual passage of the projectile through the nerve itself.

Mechanism of Recovery

When an end organ becomes denervated, reinnervation can occur in 2 ways: through collateral sprouting of intact axons or by regeneration of the injured axon.[31] In injuries where 20% to 30% of the axons are damaged, collateral sprouting is the primary mechanism of recovery. This sprouting begins in the first 4 days after injury and continues for approximately 3 to 6 months, until recovery occurs. As may be expected, an increase in motor unit size is observed and the remaining innervated muscle hypertrophies in an attempt to compensate the initial denervation of other sections of the muscle. Over time, however, the muscle eventually atrophies as fibers without innervation shrink and outpace the ability of the remaining muscle fibers to expand.[30] There are more axonal branches that sprout than the actual number of nerves that end up eventually innervating a target organ.[32] Those branches that do not receive neurotrophic factors from the target end organ undergo a pruning process and are destined to degenerate.[33,34]

In injuries affecting greater than 90% of the axon population within a nerve, axonal regeneration is the primary means for recovery.[35] To achieve full recovery, the nerve must undergo 3 main processes: wallerian degeneration (the clearing process of the distal stump), axonal regeneration, and end-organ reinnervation. Failure of any of these processes can contribute to the poor functional outcome commonly observed in patients with peripheral nerve injuries.

Wallerian Degeneration

Axons that incur traumatic damage undergo wallerian degeneration to create a microenvironment conducive for axonal regrowth and reinnervation. This process takes place within the first week after injury when the typical markers of axonal damage occur: the loss of cell membrane integrity and the breakdown of axonal cytoskeleton. Initially, swelling occurs at both ends of the damaged neuron from futile continuation of retrograde and anterograde axonal transport.[36]

Changes at the distal stump

The axonal changes at the distal end of the severed nerve eventually lead to the breakdown of the nerve stump to make way for a newly regenerating axon. The hallmark of this phase is the granular disintegration of the cytoskeleton.[37] This occurs after a sudden inflow of extracellular ions, primarily Ca^{2+} and Na^+, leads to a cascade of events resembling apoptosis, which serves to recruit macrophages using signals elaborated from Schwann cells. It has been shown that the distal nerve stump is capable of transmitting an action potential hours after transection, a fact used to study synaptic transmission and muscle function in isolated nerve-muscle preparations.[38–40] More recently, mRNA of brain-derived neurotrophic factor (BDNF) and glial cell line–derived neurotrophic factor (GDNF) were found up-regulated whereas neurotrophin-3 (NT-3) and ciliary neurotrophic factor were down-regulated in the distal stumps of transected tibial nerves. Chronically denervated distal nerve stumps maintain these changes 6 months after injury if regeneration has not occurred.[41]

Changes at the proximal stump

The changes in the proximal stump vary based on the location of the injury relative to the neuronal body and the severity of the injury. The breakdown of the proximal stump is limited and typically only progresses to the first node of Ranvier. If the site of injury is close to the neuronal body, however,

apoptosis may occur.[42] In severe injuries, the proximal portion of the nerve undergoes chromatolysis—changing the genetic motive of the cell to alter its focus to the regeneration phenotype. During this process, proteins associated with growth, such as GAP-43, tubulin, and actin, are up-regulated, and neurofilaments (involved in maintaining axonal diameter) are down-regulated.[43–45] Endogenous neuroprotectants, such as heat shock protein 27, are up-regulated perhaps to promote the survival of the damaged neuron.[46,47] When the axon eventually reaches its target organ and neuronal maturation is required, the gene expression of the neuron will revert back from a regenerative state to a maintenance state.

Schwann cells and macrophages

Schwann cells are primary mediators in triggering many of the events in wallerian degeneration and changes in their protein expression at the site of injury are key to axon regeneration. In the absence of axonal contact, Schwann cells convert to a nonmyelinating behavior—down-regulating the expression of several proteins, such as PMP22, Krox-20,[48] P0, and connexin-32.[49] Synthesis is arrested and differentiation is promoted with production of C-jun,[50] and neurotrophic factors, such as NGF and ciliary neurotrophic factor, are produced.[51] Together, these factors contribute to the formation of a pool of new Schwann cells under the protection of endogenous compounds, such as erythropoietin.[52] These changes are bolstered by mitogens released from the proximal stump neurons, such as ATP and neuregulin,[53,54] which together with acetylcholine, help mature the new Schwann cells to a myelinating phenotype.[55]

Schwann cells clear debris through phagocytosis and by recruiting macrophages.[56] This effect is dependent on the protein, MAC-2, which supports Schwann cell phagocytosis.[57] Schwann cells are also the source of monocyte chemoattractant protein-1 (MCP-1), which works to recruit macrophages.[58]

Macrophages attracted by Schwann cells rapidly arrive at the site of nerve injury[59] —a process dependent on the breakdown of the blood-nerve barrier. Macrophages also rescue the precious cholesterol in damaged nerves and produce apolipoprotein E, among other lipoproteins.[60–62] Finally, macrophages themselves produce factors that further promote Schwann cell proliferation.[60,63]

After the clearance of myelin debris, the dedifferentiated Schwann cells proliferate on the remaining endoneurial tubes of the extracellular matrix. Collectively, these are known as the bands of Büngner and the hollow tube that is formed provides a path for the regenerating axon to regrow.[64] Greater success in reinnervation from a regenerative axon is observed when the endoneurial tube is intact and neuroma formation is favored without the tube, which shrinks if unpopulated by an axon within 4 months.[30,35] The accumulation of Na^+ channels in ectopic axons unable to find tubes may result in neuropathic pain.

Nerve Regeneration

Although the alteration in the genetic expression of the neuron from a quiescent state to a regenerative state occurs concurrently with the events of wallerian degeneration, axonal regeneration itself begins after wallerian degeneration is completed.[65] At the distal tip of the proximal bud, a growth cone is formed where calcium plays a role to promote its formation.[66] Hours after injury, the growth cone sends out filapodia to sample the microenvironment. On their way to the distal nerve stump, the filopodia are initially randomly oriented but gain direction once actin and myosin expression is up-regulated within the cell body.[45,67,68]

The mobility of the growth cone depends on the presence of particular receptors in its membrane. It can be attracted or repulsed by contact-mediated or chemical means, known as neurotropism.[69,70] Examples of guidance molecules are semaphorins, ephrins, netrins, and slits. Inhibitory guidance molecules, like collapsin-1, promote growth cone collapse. Neurotrophins, like BDNF, lessen the susceptibility of growth cones promoting nerve regeneration.[71] The rate of regeneration may vary, depending on location, along the neuron in which proximal segments may see an increase of 2 mm/d to 3 mm/d whereas more distal segments may progress at a rate of 1 mm/d to 2 mm/d.

The path of the growth cone may be disrupted by scar tissue and growth cones release proteases and plasminogen activators to clear its path. This is also to clear any cell-cell or cell-matrix interactions from non-neuronal cells that are hindering its path.[66]

Schwann cells play a substantial role in promoting axonal regeneration, because they are the main source of neurotrophic factors, which generally interact with tyrosine kinase receptors to alter the gene expression profile of the neuron to promote regeneration. This message is relayed through retrograde transport.[72] NGF has a low level of expression within healthy nerves but is up-regulated in Schwann cells during injury. NGF promotes growth and proliferation of Schwann cells and is also found on the receptors of

Schwann cells lining bands of Büngner to provide tropism to the outgrowing axon.[35] Many neurotrohic factors have been discovered, with functions ranging from improving cell survival through mechanisms of apoptosis prevention, to promoting regenerating factors in the neurons and in Schwann cells (**Table 3**).[73] Furthermore, Schwann cells produce neurite-promoting factors, which are incorporated in the extracellular matrix, such as fibronectin and laminin. Growth cones use these proteins for adhesion to the basal lamina of the endoneurial tubes.[74]

Infiltrating macrophages, after phagocytosing myelin, also promote nerve regeneration through the secretion of IL-1, which induces the expression of NGF in Schwann cells and increases the NGF-receptor (NGF-R) density on Schwann cells. This feed-forward mechanism leads to the secretion of mitogens to further trigger Schwann cell proliferation.[75] Macrophages, however, also secrete IL-1 receptor antagonist, which decreases regrowth of myelinated and unmyelinated axons when applied by an implantation tube in mice with transected sciatic nerves.[76]

When the growth cone reaches the endoneurial tube, it has a better chance of reaching the end organ. Maturation must occur before the functional connection is complete. The maturation process includes remyelination, axon enlargements, and, finally, functional reinnervation. The axonal outgrowth produces ATP and acetylcholine, which promote the change of the Schwann cell phenotype from nonmyelinating to myelinating.[55]

SHORTCOMINGS FOR RECOVERY

Although peripheral nerve injuries are not life threatening, they can cause a considerable decline in patient quality of life,[77] motivating further investigation in techniques to optimize recovery. Reinnervation is not synonymous with complete functional recovery. It is the emerging understanding of this, along with the role of clinically relevant factors, that is important to improve chances for a complete functional recovery. Key elements of neuroregeneration are gap distance, wallerian degeneration, axon guidance specificity, and end-organ viability.

The presence of an intact endoneurial tube often leads to a better outcome in nerve regeneration. Thus, grade II lesions, which confer damage to the axons alone without any damage to the surrounding connective tissue, have optimal conditions for axonal regrowth. Grades III and IV lesions, however, not only have a disrupted endoneurial tube, making it difficult to form appropriate bands of Büngner, but also have increased scar

Table 3
Summary of the changes in the molecular expression in axotomized neurons after peripheral nerve injury

		Lesion	Location	References
Neurotrophic factors/receptors				
BDNF	↑	Transection	DRG	Kashiba & Senba, 1999
	↑	CCI	DRG	Obata et al, 2003
	↑	Crush	DRG	Ernfors et al, 1993
	↑	Ligation	DRG	Fukuoka et al, 2001
	↑	Transection	MN	Gu et al, 1997
	↑	Crush	DRG	Tonra et al, 1998
	↑	Spinal ligation	DRG	Shen et al, 1999
Trk receptor	=	Crush	DRG	Ernfors et al, 1993
Ret (GDNF receptor)	↑	Transection	MN	Hammarberg et al, 2000
	=	Transection	DRG	Bennett et al, 2000
GDNF family receptor (GFR) alpha2	↓	Transection	DRG	Bennett et al, 2000; Hoke et al, 2000
GFRalpha1, GFRalpha3	↑	Transection	DRG	Bennett et al, 2000
Ret and GDNFalpha1	↑	Crush	DRG/MN	Naveilhan et al, 1997
NT-3	=	Spinal ligation	DRG	Shen et al, 1999
	=	Transection	SC	Funakoshi et al,[51] 1993
TrkB	↑	Transection	MN	Hammarberg et al, 2000
	↑	Crush	SC/DRG	Ernfors et al, 1993
NGF	=	Transection	MN	Gu et al, 1997
	↑	Spinal ligation	DRG	Shen et al, 1999
NGF receptor (NGF-R)	↑	Crush	MN	Ernfors et al, 1989
16-kDa pancreatitis-associated protein (Reg-2)	↑	Transection	DRG	Averill et al, 2002
Transcriptional factors				
c-fos	↑	Transection	MN	Gu et al, 1997
	↑	Transection	DH	Kajander et al, 1996
	↑	CCI	DH	Kajander et al, 1996; and Ro et al, 2004
c-jun	↑	Transection	DRG	Jenkins & Hunt 1991; Broude et al, 1997; and Kenney & Kocsis, 1997
	↑	Crush	MN	Jenkins & Hunt, 1991
Signal transd. and activ. of transc. 3 (STAT3)	↑(A)	Transection	DRG	Qiu et al, 2005
Activating transcription factor 3 (ATF-3)	↑	Transection	MN/DRG/DH	Tsujino et al, 2000
NF-κB	↑	Transection	DH	Pollock et al, 2005
	↑(A)	PNSL/CCI	DRG	Ma & Bisby 1998
Isl 1	↑	Crush	DRG	Vogelaar et al, 2004
DRG11, LmX1 b, Pax3	=	Crush	DRG	Vogelaar et al, 2004
Others				
Tumor necrosis factor (TNF)-α receptor 1 (p55)	↑	Crush	DRG	Ohtori et al, 2004
Nectin-3	↑	Transection	MN	Zelano et al, 2006
P38 mitogen-activated protein kinase (MAPK)	↑(A)	CCI	DRG	Obata et al, 2004a
Monocyte chemoattractant protein (MCP)-1	↑	CCI	DRG/MN/DH	Zhang & De Koninck, 2006

(continued on next page)

Table 3
(continued)

		Lesion	Location	References
Fibroblast growth factor 2 (FGF-2)	↑	Ligation	DRG	Madiai et al, 2003
Glutamate transporter Excitatory amino acid carrier 1 (EAAC1)	↓	CCI	DH	Wang et al, 2006
cAMP response element binding protein (CREB)	↑(P)	CCI	DH	Miletic et al, 2004

All the injuries were performed on the sciatic nerve in murine adult animals. The changes indicated are mainly based on studies on mRNA expression or immunoreactiviy; some are based on phosphorylation (P) or activity (A). Measurements were performed in sensory neurons of dorsal root ganglia (DRG) or motoneurones (MN) of the ventral horn; in some cases, determinations were described as expression in dorsal horn (DH) or spinal cord (SC). For each molecule, references are grouped according to type of injury, because in some cases the expression varies depending on the injury model or the cell type. The arrows (↑, increase; ↓, decrease) represent up-regulation or down-regulation.

From Navarro X, Vivo M, Valero-Cabre A. Neural plasticity after peripheral nerve injury and regeneration. Prog Neurobiol 2007;82(4):163–201; with permission.

tissue formation that can be a considerable deterrent to the growth cone, leading to disorganized outgrowth.

The more distal the injury to the neuron, the more likely it is to recover. Very proximal lesions, close to the neuronal cell bodies, often trigger programmed neuronal cell death. Proximal and distal stump gap length is also negatively correlated with successful regeneration—linking the size of the injury to the fidelity of the axonal outgrowth.

During nerve recovery, the axonal outgrowth becomes remyelinated by the resident Schwann cells. This myelination is generally much thinner than normal, however, with predictable electrical consequences.[78] In a recent study using a mouse sciatic nerve crush model, it was found that axonal neuregulin-1 types I and III restored normal levels of myelination when overexpressed in transgenic mice. Unexpectedly, denervated Schwann cells also expressed neuregulin-1 type I as a paracrine/autocrine signal, suggesting that full remyelination of regenerated axons may not occur due to simply insufficient stimulation by neuronal growth factors from Schwann cells.[79]

Even if the regenerated axon is able to reach the target, maturation is only possible if the end organ is maintained. This includes the stabilization of the neuromuscular junction in cases of motoneurons.[80] The neuromuscular junction is composed of the terminal end of the motor axon, terminal Schwann cells, and the end plate of muscle fibers containing acetylcholine receptors (AChRs) (**Fig. 2**).[81] The presence of the axon provides trophic support to the end plate and a long degenerated axon leads to dispersion of AChR clusters. Agrin, a glycoprotein released by the distal nerve terminal, is suggested to be the key regulator of AChR cluster formation.[82] In agrin-deficient mutant mice, poor cluster formation and

synaptogenesis is observed after nerve injury.[83] Taken together, these data suggest that supplementing agrin at the neuromuscular junction may preserve AChR clusters and may lead to better preservation of the end organ. Aside from dispersion, AChR turnover rate increases by a factor of 10 when an axon is not present at the end plate.[84]

Muscle fibers undergo atrophy as early as 3 weeks after denervation, with collagen deposits forming in the endomysium and the perimysium. The structural architecture of the muscle and the end-plate integrity can be maintained for up to 1 year.[65,85] After 2 years, irreversible muscle fibrosis has occurred along with muscle degeneration, leading to a permanent loss of functional muscle tissue. Sensory end organs, such as pacinian corpuscles, Meissner corpuscles, and Merkel cells, can last up to 2 to 3 years, so sensory function can still be recovered even after muscle function is permanently lost.[86] The time for growth-supportive phenotypes of Schwann cells associated with target tissues is also limited.[87] Nerve transfers have been used to try to prevent denervation atrophy, but full strength and function of muscles are seldom fully recovered.[88]

EXPERIMENTAL STRATEGIES

Various models of nerve injury are used to develop viable treatments for nerve injury. In vitro models of neuronal survival include cell culture, tissue-engineered 3-D cultures, organotypic cultures, and glial cell cultures whereas in vivo models most often involve injury to the sciatic nerve of various species.

In Vitro Models

Neurons from the dorsal root ganglion are the most commonly used neurons in neuronal cell

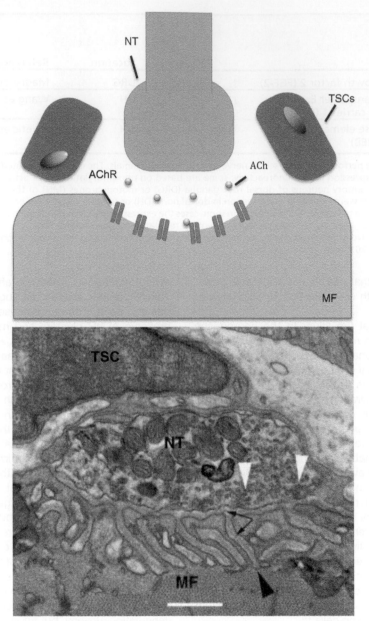

Fig. 2. The neuromuscular junction. Illustration and transition electron microscopy of the neuromuscular junction showing nerve terminal (NT), muscle fiber (MF), terminal Schwann cells (TSCs), acetylcholine (ACh), and AChRs. *White arrowheads* indicate active zones. *Black arrowhead* indicates a secondary fold. *Black arrows* indicate the basal lamina. (*From* Lee Y, Thompson WJ. The vertebrate neuromuscular junction. In: Hill JA, Olson EN, editors. Muscle: Fundamental Biology and Mechanisms of Disease. Philadelphia: Elsevier 2012; with permission.)

culture experiments. Animals only yield a small number of cells, however, which can be a prohibitive factor to using these experimental models.[89] A common cultured cell line is the rat pheochromocytoma cell line (PC12), which has neuroendocrine function and can be induced to differentiate into adult sympathetic neurons using NGF.[90] Cell cultures are commonly used for in vitro studies of the direct effects of drugs, substrates, and growth factors on neurons. Neurons cocultured with glial cells and other cell types have been useful in elucidating the interactions between those cells.

Culturing neural cells has also provided information on the dependence of neural cells on an appropriate microenvironment for optimal recovery. Tissue-engineered 3-D cultures use an artificial tissue–based extracellular matrix to study neurite growth. Contact guidance cues can be added to study axonal path taking and guidance through the endoneurial tube.[91,92] Organotypic cultures use the natural environment of the neurons in such a way that the tissue cytoarchitecture and interactions between cell types are preserved.[93,94]

In Vivo Nerve Injury Models

Animal models of crush and laceration injuries can be created to follow clinically relevant lesions and allow for greater study of molecular and cellular processes within particular nerve types (ie, mixed, motor, and sensory). Rodents are the most commonly used animals due to their inexpensive housing costs and similar distribution of nerve trunks to humans. Also, there is a large availability of genetic, cellular and systemic physiology in rodent models, including transgenic animals.[95]

The most common injury model is the sciatic nerve. Although sciatic nerve injuries in humans are rare due to the deep anatomic location within the lower extremity, animal models provide a plethora of information regarding recoveries of particular nerve types and their potential for recovery as they attempt to reach endoneurial tubules. Femoral nerve injuries in the rat are relevant in the study of particular nerve types because it has one exclusively motor branch and another that is exclusively sensory.[96,97]

Median nerve injuries are important because they are common in clinical practice, but assays of median nerve function are prohibitively difficult in rodents. Some work focuses on electrophysiologic techniques along with measures of grasping for functional outcome in rats[98] and more recently in mice using 12/0 sutures for repair after injury.[99]

Outcome Measurements of in Vivo Models

Proper outcome measurements in the assessment of functional nerve recovery are critical to defining conclusive findings. Outcome measurements include counting the number of particular structures, such as axons, neurons, reinnervated end plates, and reinnervated motor units; assessing nerve and muscle evoked potentials through electrophysiologic studies; and evaluating muscle contractile force and weight. Behavioral studies also exist particularly in assessing sciatic nerve function through walking track analysis and sensory hypersensitivity function testing. Axon count and muscle contractile forces may be the most valid assessment during the early phases of axon regeneration. At this phase, sprouts regenerate asynchronously and reach their end target at different times so may provide misleading information using evoked potentials or other forms of assessment.[100]

SUMMARY

The peripheral nerve can be injured in a variety of ways and most injuries are a mixture of various described mechanisms. The nerve can be assessed in several ways clinically but the basic and translational sciences behind new treatments are only now being elucidated. The clinical correlations of these processes when better understood promise to help guide treatment decision in the future.

REFERENCES

1. Jobe MT, Martinez SF. Peripheral nerve injuries. In: Canale ST, Beaty JH, editors. Campbell's operative orthopaedics. 12th edition. Philadelphia: Elsevier; 2013. p. 3063–5. Ch 62D.
2. Berde CB, Strichartz GR. Local anesthetics. In: Eriksson I, Fleisher LA, Wiener-Kronish JP, et al, editors. Miller's anesthesia. 7th edition. Maryland Heights, MO: Churchill Livingstone, An Imprint of Elsevier; 2009.
3. Miner JR, Paris PM, Yealy DM. Pain management. In: Marx JA, Hockberger RS, Walls RM, et al, editors. Mark Rosen's emergency medicine. 7th edition. 2010.
4. Geuna S, Raimondo S, Ronchi G, et al. Histology of the peripheral nerve and changes occurring during nerve regeneration. Int Rev Neurobiol 2009;87:27–46.
5. Rydevik B, Lundborg G. Permeability of intraneural microvessels and perineurium following acute, graded experimental nerve compression. Scand J Plast Reconstr Surg 1977;11:179–87.
6. Seddon HJ. Three types of nerve injury. Brain 1943; 66:237.
7. Sunderland S. A classification of peripheral nerve injuries producing loss of function. Brain 1951;74: 491–516.
8. Mackinnon SE, Dellon AL. Surgery of the peripheral nerve. New York: Thieme; 1988.
9. Thomas PK, Holdorff B. Neuropathy due to physical agents. In: Dyck PJ, Thomas PK, Griffin JW, editors. Peripheral neuropathy. 3rd edition. Piladelphia: W.B. Saunders; 1993. p. 990.
10. McGowan A. The results of transposition of the ulnar nerve for traumatic ulnar neuritis. J Bone Joint Surg Br 1950;32B:293–301.
11. Gupta R, Steward O. Chronic nerve compression induces concurrent apoptosis and proliferation of Schwann cells. J Comp Neurol 2003;461: 174–86.
12. Gupta R, Rummler LS, Palispis W, et al. Local down-regulation of myelin-associated glycoprotein permits axonal sprouting with chronic nerve compression injury. Exp Neurol 2006;200:418–29.

13. Ludwin SK, Maitland M. Long-term remyelination fails to reconstitute normal thickness of central myelin sheaths. J Neurol Sci 1984;64:193–8.

14. Tapadia M, Mozaffar T, Gupta R. Compressive neuropathies of the upper extremity: update on pathophysiology, classification, and electrodiagnostic findings. J Hand Surg Am 2010;35:668–77.

15. Gray M, Palispis W, Popovich PG, et al. Macrophage depletion alters the blood-nerve barrier without affecting Schwann cell function after neural injury. J Neurosci Res 2007;85:766–77.

16. Gupta R, Channual JC. Spatiotemporal pattern of macrophage recruitment after chronic nerve compression injury. J Neurotrauma 2006;23(2):216–26.

17. Frieboes LR, Gupta R. An in-vitro traumatic model to evaluate the response of myelinated cultures to sustained hydrostatic compression injury. J Neurotrauma 2009;26:2245–56.

18. O'Brien JP, Mackinnon SE, MacLean AR, et al. A model of chronic nerve compression in the rat. Ann Plast Surg 1987;19:430–5.

19. Gupta R, Nassiri N, Hazel A, et al. Chronic nerve compression alters Schwann cell myelin architecture in a murine model. Muscle Nerve 2012;45(2):231–41.

20. Diao E, Shao F, Liebenberg E, et al. Carpal tunnel pressure alters median nerve function in a dose-dependent manner: a rabbit model for carpal tunnel syndrome. J Orthop Res 2005;23:218–23.

21. Dellon AL, Mackinnon SE. Chronic nerve compression model for the double crush hypothesis. Ann Plast Surg 1991;26:259–64.

22. Molinari WJ III, Elfar JC. The double crush syndrome. In Brief. J Hand Surg Am 2013;38(4):799–801.

23. Upton AR, McComas AJ. The double crush in nerve entrapment syndromes. Lancet 1973;2:359–62.

24. Dahlin LB, Lundborg G. The neurone and its response to peripheral nerve compression. J Hand Surg Br 1990;15:5–10.

25. Wilbourn AJ, Gilliatt RW. Double-crush syndrome: a critical analysis. Neurology 1997;49:21–9.

26. Nemoto K. An experimental study on the vulnerability of peripheral nerve. J Orthop Sci 1983;57:1773–86.

27. Nemoto K, Matsumoto N, Tazaki K, et al. An experimental study on the "double crush" hypothesis. J Hand Surg Am 1987;12:552–9.

28. Dellon AL, Mackinnon SE, Seiler WA. Susceptibility of the diabetic nerve to chronic compression. Ann Plast Surg 1988;20:117–9.

29. Nishimura T, Hirata H, Tsujii M, et al. Pathomechanism of entrapment neuropathy in diabetic and nondiabetic rats reared in wire cages. Histol Histopathol 2008;23:157–66.

30. Tsao B, Boulis N, Bethoux F, et al. Trauma of the nervous system, peripheral nerve trauma. In: Daroff RB, Fenichel GM, Jankovic J, et al, editors. Bradley's neurology in clinical practice. 6th edition. 2012. p. 984–1001.

31. Zochodne DW, Levy D. Nitirc oxide in damage, disease and repair of the peripheral nervous system. Cell Mol Biol (Noisy-le-grand) 2005;51:255–67.

32. Aguayo AJ, Peyronnard JM, Bray GM. A quantitative ultrastructural study of regeneration from isolated proximal stumps of transected unmyelinated nerves. J Neuropathol Exp Neurol 1973;32:256–70.

33. Sanders FK, Young JZ. The indluence of peripheral connection on the diameter of regenerating nerve fibers. J Exp Biol 1946;22:203–12.

34. Griffin JW, Hoffman PN. Degeneration and regeneration in the peripheral nervous system. In: Dyck PJ, Thomas P, editors. Peripheral neuropathy. Philadelphia: WB Saunders; 1993.

35. Campbell WW. Evaluation and management of peripheral nerve injury. Invited review. Clin Neurophysiol 2008;119:1951–65.

36. Lunn ER, Brown MC, Perry VH. The pattern of axonal degeneration in the peripheral nervous system varies with different types of lesion. Neuroscience 1990;35:157–65.

37. George R, Griffin JW. The proximo-distal spread of axonal degeneration in the dorsal columns of the rat. J Neurocytol 1994;23(11):657–67.

38. Miledi R, Slater CR. On the degeneration of rat neuromuscular junctions after nerve section. J Physiol 1970;207(2):507–28.

39. Jones R, Vrbova G. Two factors responsible for the development of denervation hypersensitivity. J Physiol 1974;236(3):517–38.

40. Charlton MP, Atwood HL. Modulation of transmitter release by intracellular sodium in squid giant synapse. Brain Res 1977;134(2):367–71.

41. Michalski B, Bain JR, Fahnestock M. Long-term changes in neurotrophic factor expression in distal nerve stump following denervation and reinnervation with motor or sensory nerve. J Neurochem 2008;105(4):1244–52.

42. Dieu T, Johnstone BR, Newgreen DF. Genes and nerves. J Reconstr Microsurg 2005;21:179–86.

43. Tetzlaff W, Bisby MA. Neurofilament elongation into regenerating facial nerve axons. Neuroscience 1989;29(3):659–66.

44. Tetzlaff W, Alexander SW, Miller FD, et al. Response of facial and rubrospinal neurons to axotomy: changes in mRNA expression for cytoskeletal proteins and GAP-43. J Neurosci 1991;11(8):2528–44.

45. Fu SY, Gordon T. The cellular and molecular basis of peripheral nerve regeneration. Mol Neurobiol 1997;14(1–2):67–116.

46. Costigan M, Mannion RJ, Kendall G, et al. Heat shock protein 27: developmental regulation and expression after peripheral nerve injury. J Neurosci 2005;21:2051–62.

47. Lewis SE, Mannion RJ, White FA, et al. A role for HSP27 in sensory neuron survival. J Neurosci 1999;19(89):45–53.

48. Topilko P, Schneider-Maunoury S, Baron-Van Evercooren A, et al. Krox-20 controls myelination in the peripheral nervous system. Nature 1994; 371:796–9.

49. Hall S. Mechanisms of repair after traumatic injury. In: Dyck PJ, Thomas PK, editors. Peripheral neuropathy. Philadelphia: Elsevier, Saunder; 2005. p. 1403–33.

50. Parkinson DB, Bhaskaran A, Arthur-Farraj P, et al. c- Jun is a negative regulator of myelination. J Cell Biol 2008;181:625–37.

51. Funakoshi H, Friesen J, Barbany G, et al. Differential expression of mRNAs for neurotrophins and their receptors after axotomy of the sciatic nerve. J Cell Biol 1993;123:455–65.

52. Elfar JC, Jacobson JA, Puzas JE, et al. Erythropoietin accelerates functional recovery after peripheral nerve injury. J Bone Joint Surg Am 2008;90: 1644–53.

53. Pellegrino RG, Spencer PS. Schwann cell mitosis in response to regenerating peripheral axons in vivo. Brain Res 1985;341(1):16–25.

54. Birchemier C, Nave KA. Neuregulin-1 a key axonal signal that drives Schwann cell growth and differentiation. Glia 2008;56(14):1491–7.

55. Vrbova G, Mehra N, Shanmuganathan H, et al. Chemical communication between regenerating motor axons and Schwann cells in the growth pathway. Eur J Neurosci 2009;30(3):366–75.

56. Stoll G, Griffin JW, Li CY, et al. Wallerian degeneration in the peripheral nervous system: participation of both Schwann cells and macrophages in myelin degradation. J Neurocytol 1989;18:671–83.

57. Reichert F, Saada A, Rotshenker S. Peripheral nerve injury induces Schwann cells to express two macrophage phenotypes: phagocytosis and the galactose-specific lectin MAC-2. J Neurosci 1994;14:3231–45.

58. Toews AD, Barrett C, Morel P. Monocyte chemoattractant protein 1 is responsible for macrophage recruitment following injury to sciatic nerve. J Neurosci Res 1998;53:260–7.

59. Taskinen HS, Roytta M. The dynamics of macrophage recruitment after nerve transection. Acta Neuropathol 1997;82:412–25.

60. Bruck W. The role of macrophages in Wallerian degeneration. Brain Pathol 1997;7(2):741–52.

61. Rothshenker S. Microglia and macrophage activation and the regulation of complement-receptor-3 (CR3/MAC-1)-mediated myelin phagocytosis in injury and disease. J Mol Neurosci 2003;21(1): 65–72.

62. Venezie RD, Toews AD, Morell P. Macrophage recruitment in different models of nerve injury: lysozyme as a marker for active phagocytosis. J Neurosci Res 1995;40:99–107.

63. Baichwal J, Bigbee W, Devries GH. Macrophage-mediated myelin-related mitogenic factor for cultured Schwann cells. Neurobiology 1988;85: 1701–5.

64. Weinberg HJ, Spencer PS. The fate of Schwann cells isolated from axonal contact. J Neurocytol 1978;7(5):555–69.

65. Burnett MG, Zager EL. Pathophysiology of peripheral nerve injury: a brief review. Neurosurg Focus 2004;16:1–7.

66. Dahlin LB. Nerve injury and repair: from molecule to man. In: Slutsky DJ, Hentz VR, editors. Peripheral nerve surgery: practical applications in the upper extremity. Philadelphia: Churchill Livingston, Elsevier; 2006. p. 1–22.

67. Geraldo S, Gordon-Weeks PR. Cytoskeletal dynamics in growth-cone steering. J Cell Sci 2009; 122(20):3595–604.

68. Jin LQ, Zhang G, Jamison C Jr, et al. Axon regeneration in the absence of growth cones: acceleration by cyclic AMP. J Comp Neurol 2009;515(3): 295–312.

69. Marx J. Helping neurons find their way. Science 1995;268:971–3.

70. Goodman CS. Mechanisms and molecules that control growth cone guidance. Annu Rev Neurosci 1996;19:341–77.

71. Tuttle R, O'Leary DD. Neurotrophins rapidly modulate growth cone response to the axon guidance molecule, collapsin-1. Mol Cell Neurosci 1998;11: 1–8.

72. Frostick SP, Yin Q. Schwann cells, neurotrophic factors, and peripheral nerve regeneration. Microsurgery 1998;18:397–405.

73. Pham K, Gupta R. Understanding the mechanisms of entrapment neuropathies. Review article. Neurosurg Focus 2009;26(2):E7.

74. Hall S. Axonal regeneration through acellular muscle grafts. J Anat 1997;190:57–71.

75. Davis JB, Stroobant P. Platelet-derived growth factors and fibroblast growth factors are mitogens for rat Schwann cells. J Cell Biol 1990; 110:1353–60.

76. Guenard V, Dinarello CA, Weston PJ, et al. Peripheral nerve regeneration is impeded by interleukin-l receptor antagonist released from a polymeric guidance channel. J Neurosci Res 1991;29:396–400.

77. Battison B, Papalia I, Tos P, et al. Peripheral nerve repair and regeneration research: a historical note. Int Rev Neurobiol 2009;87:1–7.

78. Schröder JM. Altered ratio between axon diameter and myelin sheath thickness in regenerated nerve fibers. Brain Res 1972;45:49–65.

79. Stassart RM, Fledrich R, Velanac V, et al. A role for Schwann cell-derived neuregulin-1 in remyelination. Nat Neurosci 2013;16(1):48–54.

80. Kang JR, Zamorano DP, Gupta R. Limb salvage with major nerve injury: current management and future directions. J Am Acad Orthop Surg 2011; 19(Suppl 1):S28–34.

81. Hughes BW, Kusner LL, Kaminski HJ. Molecular architecture of the neuromuscular junction. Muscle Nerve 2006;33(4):445–61.

82. Reist NE, Werle MJ, McMahan UJ. Agrin released by motor neurons induces the aggregation of acetylcholine receptors at neuromuscular junctions. Neuron 1992;8(5):865–8.

83. Gautam M, Noakes PG, Moscoso L, et al. Defective neuromuscular synaptogenesis in agrin-deficient mutant mice. Cell 1996;85(4):525–35.

84. Shyng SL, Salpeter MM. Degradation rate of acetylcholine receptors inserted into denervated vertebrate neuromuscular junctions. J Cell Biol 1989;108(2):647–51.

85. Kline DG. Clinical and electrical evaluation. In: Kim DH, Midha R, Murovic JA, et al, editors. Kline & Hudson's nerve injuries. 2nd edition. Philadelphia: Elsevier, Saunders; 2008. p. 43–63.

86. Suzuki Y, Shirai Y. Motor nerve conduction analysis of double crush syndrome in a rabbit model. J Orthop Sci 2003;8:69–74.

87. Furey MJ, Midha R, Xu QG, et al. Prolonged target deprivation reduces the capacity of injured motoneurons to regenerate. Neurosurgery 2007;60(4):723–32.

88. Noaman HH, Shiha AE, Bahm J. Oberlin's ulnar nerve transfer to the biceps motor nerve in obstetric brachial plexus palsy: indications, and good and bad results. Microsurgery 2004;24(3):182–7.

89. Federoff S, Richardson A. Protocols for neural cell culture. Totowa (NJ): Humana Press; 2001.

90. Greene LA, Tischler AS. Establishment of a noradrenergic clonal line of rat adrenal pheochromocytoma cells which respond to nerve growth factor. Proc Natl Acad Sci U S A 1976; 73(7):2424–8.

91. Bellamkonda R, Ranieri JP, Aebischer P. Laminin oligopeptide derivatized agarose gels allows three0dimensional neurite extension in vitro. J Neurosci 1995;41:501–9.

92. Ahmed Z, Brown RA. Adhesion, alignment, and migration of cultured Schwann cells on ultrathin fibronectin fibres. Cell Motil Cytoskeleton 1999;42: 331–43.

93. Hall SM. The biology of chronically denervated Schwann cells. Ann N Y Acad Sci 1999;883: 215–33.

94. Maniwa S, Iwata A, Hirata H, et al. Effects of neurotrohic factors on chemokinesis of Schwann cells in culture. Scand J Plast Reconstr Surg Hand Surg 2003;37(1):14–7.

95. Rodriguez FJ, Valero-Cabre A, Navarro X. Regeneration and functional recovery following peripheral nerve injury. Drug Discov Today Dis Model 2004; 1(2):177–85.

96. Brushart TM, Gerber J, Kessens P, et al. Contributions of pathway and neuron preferential motor reinnervation. J Neurosci 1998;18:8674–81.

97. Madison RD, Archibald SJ, Brushart TM. Reinnervation accuracy of the rat femoral nerve by motor and sensory neurons. J Neurosci 1996; 16:5698–703.

98. Papalia I, Tos P, Stagno d'Alcontres F, et al. On the use of grasping test in the rat median nerve model: a reappraisal of its efficacy for quantitative assessment of motor function recovery. J Neurosci Methods 2003;134:75–80.

99. Tos P, Ronchi G, Nicolino S, et al. Employment of the mouse median nerve model for the experimental assessment of peripheral nerve regeneration. J Neurosci Methods 2008;169(1): 119–27.

100. Wood MD, Kemp SW, Borschel GH, et al. Outcome measures of peripheral nerve regeneration. Ann Anat 2011;193:321–33.

Nerve Allografts and Conduits in Peripheral Nerve Repair

Michael Y. Lin, MD, PhD, Givenchy Manzano, BS,
Ranjan Gupta, MD*

KEYWORDS

- Nerve conduit • Allograft • Peripheral nerve injury • Peripheral nerve repair

KEY POINTS

- Nerve repair with nerve autograft remains the gold standard for situations that preclude primary tensionless end-to-end neurorrhaphy.
- Modern processed nerve allograft requires no immune modulation and has shown promising clinical results. However valid comparison is lacking to allow meaningful comparison with nerve autograft.
- Synthetic nerve conduits are gaining popularity but its application is currently limited to small-caliber sensory nerves.
- Ongoing discoveries in neuroscience and biomaterial engineering hold promise for the development of effective nerve conduits.

INTRODUCTION

Peripheral nerve injury is a relatively common sequela of trauma with an incidence estimated between 13 and 23 per 100 persons per year.[1–3] When a nerve is transected, the goal is to perform a tensionless, primary neurorrhaphy. If a segmental nerve gap precludes such repair, the current gold standard is to bridge the nerve defect with a sensory nerve autograft. However, autologous nerve grafts are limited in supply, inherently associated with donor site morbidities, and despite the best repair techniques, frequently result in disappointing clinical outcome. For these reasons, clinicians and scientists have developed nerve allograft and conduits, encompassing both biologic and artificial materials, to serve as axonal guidance channels. These tubular structures are designed to bridge the gap of severed nerve to facilitate neuronal reconnection. Over the past 3 decades, incremental advancements have been made. Here, we review the current literature relevant to the clinical application and the evolving advancement in the design of nerve conduits and allografts for bridging segmental nerve gaps.

ANATOMY AND PATHOPHYSIOLOGY

Peripheral nerves are heterogeneous composite structures composed of fascicular bundles of axons with their cell bodies residing within and adjacent to the spinal cord. Four layers of connective tissue sheaths organize the nerve. From the outside to inward, these structures are the mesoneurium, epineurium, perineurium, and endoneurium. The mesoneurium is a connective tissue sheath that suspends the nerve trunk within the soft tissue that contains the segmental blood supply to the nerve. The epineurium is a layer of loose meshwork of collagen bundles, elastin fibers,

Disclosure: The authors have nothing to disclose.

M.Y.L and G.M. contributed equally to this work.

Department of Orthopaedic Surgery, University of California Irvine, 2226 Gillespie Neuroscience Research Facility, Irvine, CA 92697, USA

* Corresponding author.

E-mail address: ranjang@uci.edu

Hand Clin 29 (2013) 331–348

http://dx.doi.org/10.1016/j.hcl.2013.04.003

0749-0712/13/$ – see front matter Published by Elsevier Inc.

scattered fibroblasts, and adipocytes that defines the nerve trunk and provides mechanical protection. Within the nerve trunk, the perineurium is a multilayered sheath of flattened and densely packed supporting pericytes that surrounds groups of axons, and subdivides the nerve into fascicular bundles. Additionally, the perineurium is the major contributor to nerve tensile strength, serves as a diffusion barrier analogous to the blood-nerve barrier, and contains a latticework for vascular bed. The endoneurium is a loose collagenous matrix within each nerve fascicle that surrounds the individual axons and their Schwann cells.

The blood supply to the peripheral nerve is a complex vascular plexus fed by radicular vessels in the mesoneurium. Anastomotic connections between epineurial and perineurial plexi occur at various levels in the perineurium and eventually arborize into the network of endoneurial capillaries. This vascular plexus is exquisitely sensitive to tension, as animal studies have demonstrated an 80% decrease in blood flow and irreversible ischemic damage with a 15% increase in nerve tension.[4]

Despite its regenerative potential, the injured human peripheral nerve rarely spontaneously restores its function. Severing a nerve uniquely affects the entire neuron, as the recovery after nerve transaction not only requires the healing of the injury site but also necessitates the outgrowth of axons from the site of injury to the target organ for reconnection and functional recovery. Depending on the level of injury, this may require the injured nerve to regenerate very long distances, sometimes requiring many months of regeneration.

After a transaction injury, the distal nerve stump undergoes Wallerian degeneration. This cascade of events is triggered by granular disintegration of the axonal cytoskeleton at the site of injury. The initial cellular swelling is accompanied by chromatolysis and peripheral migration of nuclei. The proximal neural stump retracts, and the adjacent Schwann cells undergo apoptosis. Within 48 to 96 hours, myelin and axons begin to degrade in the distal nerve stump. At the conclusion of Wallerian degeneration, an endoneurial tube of the distal stump remains. Schwann cells then organize into Bands of Bungner[5] within the endoneurial tube. The end result is a natural "conduit" that possesses the appropriate structural scaffold and molecular cues to guide the axonal growth cone toward the target organ.

Successful functional recovery requires target organ reinnervation, which in turn is influenced by the level of injury, the age of the patient, and local biologic factors, such as the extent and severity of damage at the site of injury.[5] Because regeneration must proceed through the entire distal stump to reach the target organ, the level of injury is particularly influential in determining the eventual clinical outcome, as proximal injuries and larger nerve defects require longer regeneration time. The resulting prolonged end-organ denervation can lead to its degeneration and fibrosis.[6] Most authorities agree that poor functional recovery is expected if the growth cone fails to reinnervate the motor end plate by 12 months, citing secondary end-organ degeneration.[7,8] Until recently, evidence for the prevention of end-organ degeneration was largely lacking. A recent study provided convincing data that stabilization of the neuromuscular endplate leads to more efficient nerve regeneration in the setting of chronic denervation.[7]

HISTORY OF PERIPHERAL NERVE REPAIR

The concept of nerve repair dates back to the seventh century when Paul Aegina approximated cut nerve ends before wound closure. However, it was not until the American Civil War (1861–1865) that knowledge of peripheral nerve injuries was accumulated systematically, accelerating our understanding of nerve injury. In 1872, Neuter introduced the concept of primary repair by epineural suturing of transected nerve ends. It was quickly evident that repairs under tension hindered nerve regeneration, which led to the novel idea of bridging the nerve gap with autologous nerve grafts.[9] Initial use of non-nervous tissue conduits soon followed with the use of decalcified bone canals by Gluck in 1880 and Vanlair in 1882. The use of arterial and vein grafts as bridging conduits was introduced in the late 1800s by Bungner and in 1909 by Wrede, respectively.[8] To avoid donor site morbidity, clinicians explored the use of exogenous biologic and synthetic conduits. Although these initial efforts were met with uniformly poor results, functional efficacy was eventually observed in the late 1980s with the advent of immune suppression for nerve allografts and the development of silicone and polyglycolic acid in the case of nerve conduits.[10,11] Because detailed understanding of the biology of regenerating nerves was unavailable, much of the work on nerve conduits in the past 3 decades relied on empiric evidence and "common sense" logic. However, despite these limitations, impressive progress was achieved.

ALLOGRAFT

Albert[9] was the first to describe the use of nerve allograft in 1885, but reported poor clinical results.

Subsequent studies pointed to immune rejection as the likely cause of host-mediated scarring and fibrosis[12] that led to clinical failure.[13,14] In the second half of the twentieth century, host immunosuppression was developed, which allowed nerve allotransplantation to become a possible reconstructive option. Additionally, a series of analysis on nerve regeneration through nerve allograft led to the conclusion that immune suppression may be stopped once regeneration is complete and end-organ connections are reestablished.[15–17] It was speculated that immunosuppressed allografts functioned as a structural scaffold for regenerating host nerve fibers. As regeneration proceeds, donor antigenic determinants within the allograft, such as Schwann cells, are lost and replaced by host components.[16,18] This concept of allografting with a limited period of immunosuppression was applied clinically in 2001, when Mackinnon and colleagues[19] reconstructed large peripheral nerve gaps in 7 patients with nerve allografts pretreated to decrease graft immunogeneity. Patients then received immunomodulation with cyclosporine A or tacrolimus and prednisone until 6 months after regeneration was evident. In this series, 6 patients demonstrated return of motor function and sensation in the affected limb, and only 1 patient experienced rejection secondary to subtherapeutic immunosuppression.

Efforts to completely eliminate immunosuppression led to the development of decellularized nerve allografts (**Table 1**). These processed human nervous tissues have reduced immunogenicity and thereby preclude the need for immune modulation, yet allowed the graft to retain many of the beneficial characteristics of a nerve graft. These include the physical macrostructure, the extracellular matrix (ECM), and associated scaffolding that may facilitate nerve regeneration.[19–23] Methods to decellularize allografts include irradiation, freeze thawing, detergent-processing, and cold preservation. AxoGen processing is a proprietary combination of decellularization methods producing the only commercially available allograft currently approved by the Food and Drug Administration (FDA) for clinical use.

The decellularization process alters the molecular and structural properties a nerve. In fact, Moore and colleagues[24] bridged a 14-mm rat sciatic nerve defect with rat nerves processed via different methods to determine whether the decellularization process influenced the functional outcome. They showed that allograft processed with detergent had similar performance to isografts and superior performance to allografts prepared by either cold preservation or AxoGen

processing. It was theorized that detergent processing required shorter times and possibly allowed retention of growth factors released from the ECM.[24] In humans, allograft has shown promising outcomes in peripheral nerve repair.[21,25,26] When compared with conduits, decellularized allografts were superior in regeneration and function[27] and perhaps equivalent to autografts in selected situations. This difference may stem from the retention of Schwann cell basal lamina and ECM scaffolding.

An interesting potential modification of nerve allograft involves the concept of "predegeneration." As detailed previously, the natural course of the transacted distal nerve stump is the formation of a native neural tube lined with Bands of Bungner through the process of Wallerian degeneration. This degeneration process was hypothesized to be a necessary prerequisite before growth cone entry into the nerve graft and is referred to as predegeneration. Base on this logic, a nerve graft may be rendered favorable for nerve regeneration more quickly if appropriate processing could be performed (in vivo or in vitro) before implantation, thus potentially shortening the delay time for nerve regeneration.[28,29] However, whether predegeneration definitively enhances the effectiveness of nerve allografts remains unanswered. In animal studies, Trumble[30] found that predegenerated allografts demonstrated better neurologic recovery compared with standard allografts; however, Dubuisson and colleagues[31] demonstrated that predegeneration of allografts resulted in larger mean nerve fiber diameter but produced no difference in myelinated nerve fiber density, electromyography, nerve conduction velocity, or nerve action potential amplitude at 2 and 3 months. One challenge with predegeneration is the uncertainty over the optimal time required for the process of predegeneration before repair. Available evidence implicates beneficial effect with as little as 1 day of in vivo predegeneration,[29] whereas 15 weeks of predegeneration began to impede nerve regeneration.[32] Current thinking favors 4 weeks as the optimal predegeneration period, as it allows full debris elimination,[33,34] enhanced collagen production,[35] peak Schwann cell proliferation,[36] and upregulation of trophic and adhesive factors that facilitate nerve growth.[37,38]

Along similar logic to in vivo predegeneration of nerve grafts, in vitro modification of allograft can facilitate the degradation of chrondroitin sulfate proteoglycans (CSPGs), a molecule present in distal nerve stumps and an implicated inhibitor of axonal growth.[39] The addition of chondroitinase ABC (cABC), a CSPG degrading enzyme, to freeze thawed allografts, has been shown to enhance

Table 1
Clinical studies for nerve allograft

Reference	Nerve Injured	Gap, mm	Conduit Material	Comparison	Mean Follow-up Time, mo	Functional Outcomes			Level of Evidence
						S4 <6 mm s2pd	S3+ 7–15 mm s2pd	S3–S0 >15 mm s2pd	
Karabekmez et al,[21] 2009	Digital nerves and sensorial branches of ulnar nerve	22.3 (5–30)	Allograft	None	9 (5–12)	5/10 (50%)	5/10 (50%)	0/10 (0%)	Level 4: prospective observation
Brooks et al,[25] 2012	Digital nerves (60%), upper extremity nerves (32%), head and neck (5%), lower extremity (3%)	22 (5–50)	Allograft	None	8.8 ± 5.1	*Reported as meaningful recovery S4/S3+ in %.* Overall: 87% Nerve type: Sensory (88.6%), mixed (77%), motor (85.7%), $P > .05$ Gap size: 5–14 mm (100%), 15–29 mm (76.25), 30–50 mm (95.5%), $P > .05$ Time of repair: Acute (87.1%), delayed (100%), chronic (83.3%), $P > .05$ Age: 18–29 (70%), 30–49 (88.2%), 50–86 (92.9%), $P > .05$ Injury type: Laceration (88.9%), neuroma resection (87.5%), complex (81.8%), $P > .05$			Level 4: prospective observation
Cho et al,[26] 2012	Digital, median, ulnar with sensory, mixed, motor	23 ± 12 (5–50)	Allograft	None	Not reported	*Reported as meaningful recovery S4/S3+ in %.* Nerve type: Sensory (86%), motor (80%), $P > .05$ Gap length: 5–14 mm (100%), 15–29 (74%), 30–50 (90%), $P > .05$ Nerve involved: Digital (89%), median (75%), ulnar (67%)			Level 4: retrospective case review

Abbreviations: S2PD, static 2 point discrimination; S4, excellent recovery; S3+, good recovery; S3–S0, poor nerve recovery.

axonal regeneration and functional outcomes in animals.[40] It was suggested that cABC enhanced the adhesive properties of the allograft basal lamina, thus promoting nerve regeneration.[41] The incorporation of cABC into AxoGen-processed allografts represents an application of biologic knowledge to clinical practice, and spurred much enthusiasm for AxoGen allografts. In 2012, Brooks and colleagues[25] performed a multicenter outcome study in which nerve defects between 5 and 50 mm were repaired with AxoGen grafts. Analysis showed meaningful recovery (S3+/S4 or M4/M5) in 87% of patients. Subgroup analysis demonstrated a higher rate of recovery in the sensory group compared with the mixed and motor only groups (P>.05). In the same year, Cho and colleagues[26] also reported on the use of AxoGen allografts for sensory, mixed, and motor nerve gaps of 5 to 50 mm. An overall 86% meaningful recovery was observed. Subgroup analysis revealed meaningful recovery in 89% of digital nerve repairs, 75% of median nerve repairs, and 67% of ulnar nerve repairs. Subgroup analysis on nerve type (ie, sensory, mixed, or motor) demonstrated an 86% and 80% meaningful recovery for sensory and motor nerves respectively (P>.05). Although these results compared favorably to prior investigations for nerve autograft, it is difficult to draw a meaningful conclusion on the allograft's efficacy because valid comparison to nerve autograft is lacking. Additionally, the high distribution of digital sensory nerves must be critically accounted for when considering the observed high rate of recovery (see **Table 1**).

Despite the growing clinical popularity, recent animal studies suggest that allografts may still be inferior to fresh autografts in the ability to support nerve regeneration.[27]

CONDUITS
Autologous Conduits

The use of autologous non-neuronal tissue as conduits was first reported in 1891 when Bungner[42] demonstrated successful sciatic nerve regeneration through a segment of human brachial artery. Although studies on regeneration through arterial grafts continued through the twentieth century,[43–45] the high morbidity and lack of dispensable donor vessels have rendered arterial grafts less popular than alternatives in nerve repair. However, it was recently shown that injuries to the neurovascular bundle in the hand might benefit from the use of injured homolateral arteries for repair of associated segmental nerve defects.

Veins have also been a viable option for nerve repair. Proponents cite their abundant supply and minimal donor morbidity as advantages over arterial grafts. Wrede was the first to bridge a median nerve gap with a 45-mm vein graft.[46,47] Subsequent studies demonstrated meaningful recovery when vein grafts were used to bridge digital sensory nerve gaps of 3 cm or smaller.[48,49] Recently, Rinker and Liau[50] demonstrated similar sensory recovery when nerve gaps of 4 to 25 mm were repaired with either vein graft or collagen conduits, with vein grafts yielding fewer complications. Although vein conduits have shown potential for nerve repair, opponents are concerned with the possibility of lumen collapse possibly impeding nerve regeneration.[51]

Efforts to limit the risk of vein collapse led to the filling of vein grafts with nerve or muscle tissue. These intraluminal additives have theoretical benefits of supplying neurotrophic factors (nervous tissue) and ECM (muscle fibers), and have been theorized to facilitate nerve regeneration across longer gaps by promoting Schwann cell migration, cell proliferation, and guidance of the axonal growth cone.[52,53] Veins with interposed neuronal tissue have been shown to produce meaningful recovery in ulnar, median, digital, and superficial radial nerve defects of 2.5 to 4.5 cm.[54,55] Likewise, superior functional and histologic outcomes have been demonstrated with combined vein–muscle conduits compared with muscle grafts alone, but with limitations to gaps of 2 cm or smaller.[56] However, attempts to achieve functional recovery over larger sensory and mixed nerve gaps larger than 2 cm have been more difficult to achieve.[57] Although some positive outcomes have been demonstrated, the superiority of filled vein conduits to autograft has not been established.

Another biologic conduit of historical interest is the tendon autograft. Its anisotropicity, ECM macrostructure, and presence of hyaluronic acid possessed a theoretical beneficial effect on the regenerating nerve cone.[58] Proponents also cited additional benefits, such as the abundance of donor grafts and limited loss of function from donor sites.[59] Early studies to bridge the neural gap with autologous tendons demonstrated positive outcomes in 1.0-cm defects of the rabbit deep peroneal nerve and rat sciatic nerve[60,61] and in 1.5-cm defects of the rat sciatic nerve.[62] Insight into the importance of Schwann cells in nerve regeneration prompted further studies involving pretreatment of autologous tendon with segments of injured nerve or seeding of grafts with Schwann cells before grafting in animal studies.[60,62] With both treatments, enhanced nerve regeneration was observed compared with either non-pretreated or nonseeded grafts. These preclinical studies illustrate the feasibility of bridging the neural gap with tendon autografts. However, with the absence of clinical studies, it remains uncertain whether autologous tendons are useful in human nerve repair.

Synthetic Conduits

The earliest success with synthetic conduits was observed in 1989 by Merle and colleagues,[10] who bridged nerve defects with silicone nerve guides. Lundborg and colleagues[63–65] later published multiple case reports illustrating the feasibility of silicone conduits for nerve repair. However, despite these early promising results, the nonresorbable nature of silicone caused permanent fibrotic encapsulation of the implant with subsequent chronic nerve compression. Not only was nerve regeneration impeded, patients often required secondary surgical interventions.[66] These limitations have made silicone conduits obsolete and led to the development of absorbable synthetic conduits.

Intensive studies since the early 1990s have led to the development of 3 types of synthetic conduits that are FDA approved: polyglycolic acid (PGA), collagen type 1, and caprolactone. Currently, the use of synthetic nerve conduits have been limited to gaps 3 cm or smaller in small-caliber sensory digital nerves. However, with advances in bioengineering, there is increasing potential for extending clinical applications of synthetic conduits to the repair of larger nerve defects.[67]

PGA

PGA is a commonly used suture material and was the first material used to construct nerve conduits when the limitations of silicon tubes were noted. It has excellent mechanical properties and is rapidly degraded into lactic acid in 90 days. Critics remain concerned that PGA may be degraded before completion of nerve regeneration, whereas others focus on the possible toxic affects of its lactic acid degradation product.

Despite these criticisms, PGA conduits have yielded positive outcomes in both sensory and motor segmental nerve gaps (**Table 2**). Early success with PGA was noted by Mackinnon and Dellon,[68] who performed a case series of 15 secondary reconstructions of digital nerve defects 3 cm or smaller with PGA conduits and reported an 86% meaningful recovery. Efforts to extend the use of PGA to larger defects and motor nerves were undertaken by Rosson and colleagues,[67] who bridged median nerve defects of 15 to 40 mm and reported meaningful motor recovery in all patients. Although these studies demonstrate the feasibility of PGA conduits to bridge a variety of nerve defects, they do not make any

direct comparisons with conventional repair with autograft.

In an attempt to address this deficiency, Weber and colleagues[69] conducted a randomized prospective multicenter trial comparing the efficacy of PGA tubes to nerve autografting or end-to-end repair. Gaps repaired averaged 7 mm for the PGA group and 4.3 mm for the standard repair group. After 12 months, 74% meaningful recovery was noted in the PGA group compared with 86% in the standard techniques group ($P>.05$). Subgroup analysis by gap length showed superior sensory recovery in gaps of less than 4 mm and 9 to 30 mm when the repair was performed with PGA conduit compared with end-to-end repair or autograft, respectively ($P<.05$).[69]

Subsequent studies comparing PGA to nonneuronal methods of nerve repair found PGA to perform equally or better. In 2005, Battiston and colleagues[70] compared PGA conduits and vein grafts filled with muscle fibers to repair digital nerves. Gaps in the PGA group were in the range of 1.0 to 4.0 cm, and 0.5 to 1.5 cm in the muscle-filled vein group. Meaningful recovery was noted in 94% of the PGA group and 100% of the combined muscle-vein group ($P>.05$). Subgroup analysis of age effect found no significant differences in functional outcomes in either group. In 2011, Rinker and Liau[50] performed a comparative study of PGA conduits and autogenous vein grafts for short (<10 mm) and long (≥10 mm) digital nerve gaps and found no difference in meaningful recovery between either the short-gap or long-gap cohorts.

Collagen conduits

Collagen conduits are made from highly purified type 1 collagen derived from bovine deep flexor tendons. The use of collagen is believed to facilitate adhesion and survival and enhance cell proliferation. Degradation of collagen conduits requires 48 months and this relatively long duration poses the theoretical risk of fibrosis and ensuing nerve compression.

Clinical studies evaluating the efficacy of collagen conduits have demonstrated favorable functional outcomes in sensory nerve defects of 20 mm or less (**Table 3**). In a retrospective study, Bushnell and colleagues[71] demonstrated a meaningful recovery rate of 89% in digital sensory nerves 20 mm or smaller repaired with collagen conduits. Similarly, Wangensteen and Kalliainen,[72] in a retrospective review, reported an overall 35% recovery of quantitative nerve function when collagen conduits were used for sensory nerve gaps of 2.5 to 20 mm. Lohmeyer and colleagues[73] performed a prospective cohort study in 2009 and demonstrated meaningful recovery in 75% of patients who had digital and palmar nerve gaps of 6 to 18 mm. In 2010, Thomsen and colleagues[74] performed a retrospective study of patients with painful neuroma who underwent repair with collagen conduits. Among the 11 common digital nerves repaired, meaningful recovery was seen in 5 patients. In 2011, Taras and colleagues[75] reported a 73% meaningful recovery in 5-mm to 15-mm isolated digital nerve lacerations repaired with collagen conduits. These results suggest that collagen conduits may be safe for sensory gaps of 20 mm or less, but do not confirm whether collagen is more beneficial than nerve autograft or hold any benefit for bridging larger neural gaps.

Poly D, L lactide-co-epsilon-caprolactone conduits (PCL)

PCL nerve guides are the most recent FDA-approved synthetic conduits. These have the advantage of being transparent and produce a less-acidic degradation product and therefore are theoretically less toxic to the surrounding tissue. However, the higher rigidity of PCL conduits renders them more difficult to handle in the clinical setting.

Efforts to assess the efficacy of PCL conduits have yielded mixed outcomes (**Table 4**). In a randomized prospective multicenter study by Bertleff and colleagues,[76] PCL conduits were comparable to either primary end-to-end repair or nerve autograft in 3 groups stratified by neural gap length (≤4 mm, 5–8 mm, and 9–20 mm). However, later investigations by Meek and colleagues[77] and Hernandez Cortez and colleagues[78] demonstrated no meaningful recovery when PCL conduits were used to repair digital nerves. Similarly, Chiriac and colleagues[79] performed a case series of 28 nerve repairs of the upper extremity with PCL conduits and reported only a 25% meaningful recovery with a 35% complication rate. With these conflicting results, the efficacy of PCL conduits remains unclear.

Fibrin

Interest in the use of fibrin glue for nerve repair stems from several unique properties of the liquid matrix. First, the material can be manipulated into aligned hydrogel and shaped into a tubular conduit. Second, fibrin glue is known to promote angiogenesis,[80] stimulate chemotaxis and leukocytosis, and enhance macrophage proliferation. Third, when used as an adjunct to suture repair, the solidified semisolid hydrogel provides the added benefit of hemostasis, and enhances the integrity of repair.[81] Additionally, animal studies implicate less inflammation and fibrosis when end-to-end nerve repair is performed with fibrin glue compared with suture repair. When used as a conduit, fibrin has been shown to produce equal or superior functional outcome to poly-3-hydroxybutyrate (PHB) conduits[82] or autografts.[83]

Despite favorable outcomes in preclinical investigations, clinicians remain cautious about using fibrin for nerve repair partly because of inconsistent reports of repair site tensile strength[84–86] and concerns that fibrin glue may inhibit nerve regeneration.[87] However, a recent report by Rafijah and colleagues[88] suggests that fibrin glue does not impede nerve regeneration. In fact, this was reinforced when a 10-mm rat sciatic nerve defect was repaired with collagen conduits filled with fibrin glue. At 12 weeks, although autografts continued to demonstrate superiority over collagen conduits, no difference with regard to function, axonal regeneration, and compound motor action potential was detected between normal collagen conduit and those filled with fibrin glue. These results suggest that fibrin glue may serve as an adjuvant to nerve repair and more studies should be performed to further characterize fibrin glue's efficacy for improving nerve regeneration in the clinical setting.

OPTIMIZING NERVE REGENERATION

Although current conduits have yet to reach similar efficacy as nerve autograft, the development of a new generation of conduits is under way that holds promise to dramatically enhance the efficacy of conduit-mediated nerve regeneration. These new developments aim to optimize the regenerative environment through vascularization, incorporating molecular and cell-based therapies, and architectural and surface modifications. Furthermore, recent advances in neuroscience and biomaterial engineering have gained significant insight into the molecular basis of growth cone guidance and promise to revolutionize the design of nerve conduits.

Vascularization of Grafts and Conduits

The reestablishment of blood flow to nerve grafts has long been implicated as a crucial process in successful nerve regeneration[89]; however, its precise role in nerve regeneration remains unclear.[90–95] Revascularization is especially challenging in conduits, where no preexisting blood supply exists, and in allografts, where the potential of immune inflammatory response compounds the challenge of revascularization. These challenges have led to various modalities aimed at promoting vascularization in grafts and conduits.

Table 2
Clinical studies for polyglycolic acid (PGA) conduits

Reference	Nerve Injured	Gap, mm	Conduit Material	Comparison	Mean Follow up Time, mo	Sensibility Outcomes S4 <6 mm s2pd	S3+ 7–15 mm s2pd	S3–S0 >15 mm s2pd	Level of Evidence
Rinker & Liau,[50] 2011	Digital nerves	PGA: 9.1 ± 4.6 Vein: 10.3 ± 4.8	PGA	Autogenous vein conduit	6, 12	Short gap <10 mm 6 mo: (PGA)7.3 ± 1.5 (Vein)7.7 ± 1.6, $P>.05$ 12 mo: (PGA)6.9 ± 1.7 (Vein)6.3 ± 2.0, $P>.05$ Long gap ≥10 mm 6 mo: (PGA)9.6 ± 1.9 (Vein)9.3 ± 1.9, $P>.05$ 12 mo: (PGA)8.5 ± 1.9 (Vein)8.5 ± 2.5, $P>.05$			Level 1: prospective randomized
Rosson et al,[67] 2009	Ulnar, median, spinal accessory	28 (15–40)	PGA	None	39 (4–66)	No s2pd reported. However 100% ≥M3 motor recovery			Level 4: retrospective chart review
Donoghoe et al,[133] 2007	Median nerve	30	PGA	None	24	Case 1: 2pd was S3+ in thumb, index, and middle digits Case 2: 2pd was S4 in thumb and middle digits and S3+ in index			Level 4: retrospective case series
Dellon et al,[134] 2006	Radial sensory and volar digital nerve of hallux	25	PGA	None	30	1/1 (100%)	0%	0%	Level 5: case report
Battiston et al,[70] 2005	Digital nerve	PGA: 22.6 (10–40) Vein w/muscle: 10.5 (5–15)	PGA	Vein conduit with muscle filler	6–74	PGA: 13/17 (76.5%) Vein w/muscle: 10/13 (76.9%)	PGA: 3/17 (17.7%) Vein w/muscle: 3/13 (23.2%)	PGA: 1/17 (5.8%) Vein w/muscle: 0/13 (0%)	Level 3: case series with control

Study	Nerve	Conduit	Comparison						Level
Weber et al,[69] 2000	Digital nerve	PGA	Primary end-to-end and autograft	PGA: 9.4 ± 4.4 Standard: 8.1 ± 5.0	PGA: 7.0 ± 5.6 End-to-end/Autograft: 4.3 ± 6.7	Overall: PGA: 20/46 (43.5%) Control: 24/56 (42.8%) P>.05 Gap <4 mm PGA: 10/11 (91%) Control: 19/39 (49%) P<.05 Gap 5–7 mm: PGA: 17% Control: 57% P>.05 Gap >8 mm: PGA: 42% Control: 0% P>.05	Gap <4 mm PGA: 9% Control: 42% P<.05 Gap 5–7 mm: PGA: 44% Control: 29% P>.05 Gap >8 mm: PGA: 29% Control: 70% P>.05	Gap <4 mm PGA: 0% Control: 10% P<.05 Gap 5–7 mm: PGA: 39% Control: 14% P>.05 Gap >8 mm: PGA: 29% Control: 30% P>.05	Level 1: prospective multicenter randomized controlled trial
Mackinnon & Dellon,[68] 1990	Digital nerves	PGA	None	22.4 (11–32)	17(5–30)	5/15 (33%)	8/15 (53%)	2/15 (13.3%)	Level 4: prospective observational

Abbreviations: S2PD, static 2 point discrimination; S4, excellent recovery; S3+, good recovery; S3-S0, poor nerve recovery.

Table 3
Clinical studies for collagen conduits

Reference	Nerve Injured	Gap, mm	Conduit Material	Comparison	Mean Follow-up Time, mo	Sensibility Outcomes S4 <6 mm s2pd	S3+ 7–15 mm s2pd	S3-S0 >15 mm s2pd	Level of Evidence
Taras et al,[75] 2011	Digital nerves	12 (5–17)	Neuragen	None	20 (12–59)	13/22 (59%)	3/22 (13.6%)	6/22 (27.3%)	Level 4: prospective observational
Thomsen et al,[74] 2010	Digital nerves	11.25 (5–20)	Revolnerve (Porcine type 1/3 collagen)	Contralateral finger	11.8 (6–17)	4/11 (36.3%)	1/11 (9.1%)	6/11 (54.5%)	Level 4: retrospective chart review
Wangensteen et al,[72] 2010	Digital and nondigital upper extremity	2.5–20; ± 11.7/12.8	Neuragen	None	Not reported	2PD: 24% improvement SW: 67% improvement EMG: 33% improvement			Level 4: retrospective chart review
Lohmeyer et al,[73] 2009	Digital nerves repairs	12.5 ± 3.7	Neuragen	None	12	4/12 (33%)	5/12 (42%)	3/12 (25%)	Level 2: prospective cohort
Bushnell et al,[71] 2008	Digital nerve	<20 mm	Neuragen	None	15 (12–22)	4/9 (44%)	4/9 (44%)	1/9 (11.1%)	Level 4: retrospective review

Abbreviations: EMG, electromyography; S2PD, static 2 point discrimination; S4, excellent recovery; S3+, good recovery; S3-S0, poor nerve recovery; SW, Semmes-Weinstein monofilament testing.

Table 4
Clinical studies for caprolactone conduits

Reference	Nerve Injured	Gap, mm	Conduit Material	Comparison	Mean Follow-up Time, mo	Sensibility Outcomes				Level of Evidence
						S4 <6 mm s2pd	S3 + 7–15 mm s2pd	S3–S0 >15 mm s2pd		
Bertleff et al,[76] 2005	Digital	<20	Caprolactone	End-to-end	12	No definite values reported; however, concluded that caprolactone group was as good as control.				Level 1: Blind, randomized multicenter
Chiriac et al,[79] 2012	Upper extremity nerves in arm, elbow, forearm, wrist, palms, fingers	11.03	Caprolactone	Contralateral side	21.9 (3–45)	No 2pd performed. Weber test showed 18.89 mm difference between experimental and control sides. Semmes-Weinstein testing showed 46.92 g difference between experimental and control sides				Level 3: prospective observational with control

Abbreviations: S2PD, static 2 point discrimination; S4, excellent recovery; S3+, good recovery; S3–S0, poor nerve recovery.

One approach to promoting vascularization in grafts is prefabrication. The aim of this method is to induce vascularization by temporarily attaching nerves to a vascular carrier, such as a nearby muscle or vascular pedicle. This process has yielded mixed outcomes. In 2002, Saray and colleagues[96] implanted a free peripheral nerve graft onto an arteriovenous pedicle and demonstrated vascularization in the nerve graft with preservation of Schwann cells and nerve architecture. Subsequently, Serel and colleagues[97] implanted rat sciatic nerves onto femoral vessels and reported vascularization, but with severe nerve scarring, degeneration, and absence of measurable compound action potentials. Therefore, despite positive histologic outcomes, the lack of encouraging preclinical functional results precludes the application of prefabrication in the clinical setting.

Current efforts to encourage vascularization of conduits rely on using favorable material and incorporating growth factors that promote angiogenesis. Available evidence suggests that collagen can enhance neovascularization compared with silicone conduits.[98] The potential of enhancing vascularization with growth factors was shown recently when Hobson[99] demonstrated enhanced angiogenesis with a 17% recovery of gastrocnemius muscle weight with silicone tubes supplemented with vascular endothelial growth factor to bridge a 10-mm rat sciatic nerve defect.

Chitosan

New polymers are under investigation for use as nerve conduits. One such candidate is a chitosan-based conduit. Because of its favorable biocompatibility, biodegradability, and bioactivity, chitosan has been touted as a good biomaterial with a wide range of biomedical applications.[100] Its affinity for nerve cells and ability to promote the survival and neurite outgrowth in vitro suggests that chitosan might be applicable as a scaffold for axonal regeneration in peripheral nerves.[8] A recent case study demonstrated that repair of a 30-mm defect in the median nerve of the distal right forearm resulted in regained thumb abduction and thumb-index opposition, as well as meaningful sensory recovery.[101]

Current Developments: Molecular and Cell-Based Therapy

Prior studies have implicated an important role for Schwann cells in mediating nerve regeneration.[102] As such, Schwann cells have been seeded onto synthetic conduits to improve nerve regeneration.[103–108] Similarly, recent enthusiasm and availability of stem cells have prompted investigations on seeding stem cells to synthetic conduits as a means to improve the effectiveness of nerve conduits. Multiple types of stem cells have been used, including mesenchymal stem cells,[109] adipose tissue–derived stem cells,[110] and dental pulp stem cells. Early preclinical studies are promising, as the stem cells have ability to differentiate into neuronal-like cells,[111–115] and release favorable growth factors.[116–118] A Schwann and stem cell cocultured system has also been explored to facilitate the differentiation of stem cells with Schwann cell released growth.[119] Early animal studies suggest superior outcome when these cocultures are incorporated into nerve conduits.[119]

Aside from cell-based therapies, the addition of growth factors to conduits has also shown promise in promoting axonal regrowth.[120–122] Early experiences with growth factor–seeded conduits demonstrated improved histologic nerve regeneration, but poor functional outcomes.[123] However, the development of systems capable of controlling the release kinetics of growth factor now show promise in enhancing the effectiveness of nerve conduits. Various modalities of controlled growth factor release have been investigated. These include cross-linking of collagen[124] and fibrin-based matrix scaffolds.[125,126]

Another promising development involves tissue engineering, which allows alterations in the properties of the synthetic conduit. Current efforts focus on altering parameters, such as the geometric configuration, biocompatibility, porosity, degradation kinetics, electrical conductivity, and mechanical strength of the synthetic conduits.

Structural Modulation and Engineered Culture Substrates

The application of nanofiber internal scaffolds and surface micropatterning are newer bioengineering techniques that impart anisotropicity to synthetic conduits and have the potential to mimic the hierarchical structure of the ECM conducive to cell attachment/migration, signal transduction, and nutrient support.[127] Recent advances in engineering now allow detailed studies on the effects of altering spatial distribution of various molecules on the migration growth cone. Animal studies with nanofiber scaffolds have demonstrated improved functional recovery across the rat sciatic nerve gap when compared with either autograft[128] or an empty conduit control.[129] Studies evaluating the efficacy of micropatterned nerve conduits have also shown improved functional outcome, with recovery seen across critical length defects when compared with autograft.[130]

Future Developments: Intelligent Design Stemming from Advances in Molecular and Cellular Biology

Current evidence suggests that the growth cone of a regenerating axon is a motile structure sensitive to environmental cues. During regeneration, it behaves similarly to growth cones of a developing axon, interacting with its immediate environment by extending and retracting fingerlike projections known as filopodia and lamellipodia. The extent and direction of growth cone migration is in turn influenced by the molecular cues encountered by the probing filopodia and lamellipodia. Contact with permissive cues leads to stabilization of the involved filopodia, whereas contact with an inhibitory cue causes retraction and destabilization of its associated cytoskeleton. Recent experiments have identified several families of anchored and secreted molecules capable of modulating the behavior of the growth cone.[131] Although the emerging picture indicates complex interactions between the growth cone and guidance molecules,[132] with further understanding, it should be possible to incorporate appropriate types and concentrations of molecules into the nerve conduit to facilitate nerve growth toward its target.

SUMMARY

The goal of peripheral nerve repair is to restore normal function. Despite the advances in conduits and allografts, the application of surgical techniques for repair of peripheral nerve injuries only mechanically sets the stage for orderly progression of healing. The ultimate repair and regeneration is a complex biologic process that we are just beginning to understand.

Currently, primary tensionless end-to-end neurorrhaphy and nerve autografting continue to be the gold standards for nerve repair. Although there has been significant preclinical data to support the use of a variety of nerve conduits and allografts, the lack of well-designed, randomized control studies make it difficult to compare the efficacy of these techniques to standard repair methods. Although an abundance of observational clinical studies exist, most are performed at single institutions, with variable follow-up times, and/or lack of a standardization of the measured functional outcome. As such, limited insights may be derived from these reports.

Although broad conclusions have been drawn using data gathered from animal studies, these conclusions must be interpreted with caution because animals can achieve histomorphometric and functional recovery in injury paradigms that are insurmountable by humans.[27] For example, rodent nerves can spontaneously regenerate through an unfilled 4.5-cm nerve gap in 5 months,[27] whereas a fully transected nerve in a human must be surgically repaired for any recovery to occur.

Nerve conduits and allografts are viable alternatives that allow surgeons to avoid autograft-associated morbidities. Through better-designed studies, it may be possible to eventually stratify the effectiveness of autograft, allograft, and nerve conduits. With the combination of increasing proficiency in nerve biology and continued breakthroughs in microfabrication techniques, we are now poised to revolutionize the design of nerve conduits.

REFERENCES

1. Noble J, Munro CA, Prasad VS, et al. Analysis of upper and lower extremity peripheral nerve injuries in a population of patients with multiple injuries. J Trauma 1998;45(1):116–22.
2. Evans GR. Peripheral nerve injury: a review and approach to tissue engineered constructs. Anat Rec 2001;263(4):396–404.
3. Asplund M, Nilsson M, Jacobsson A, et al. Incidence of traumatic peripheral nerve injuries and amputations in Sweden between 1998 and 2006. Neuroepidemiology 2009;32(3):217–28.
4. Clark WL, Trumble TE, Swiontkowski MF, et al. Nerve tension and blood flow in a rat model of immediate and delayed repairs. J Hand Surg Am 1992;17(4):677–87.
5. Lee SK, Wolfe SW. Peripheral nerve injury and repair. J Am Acad Orthop Surg 2000;8(4):243–52.
6. Daly W, Yao L, Zeugolis D, et al. A biomaterials approach to peripheral nerve regeneration: bridging the peripheral nerve gap and enhancing functional recovery. J R Soc Interface 2012;9(67):202–21.
7. Chao T, Frump D, Lin M, et al. Matrix metalloproteinase 3 deletion preserves denervated motor endplates after traumatic nerve injury. Ann Neurol 2013;73(2):210–23.
8. Konofaos P, Ver Halen JP. Nerve repair by means of tubulization: past, present, future. J Reconstr Microsurg 2013;29(3):149–64.
9. Albert E. Einige operationen am nerven, vol. 26. Wien Med Press; 1885. p. 1285.
10. Merle M, Dellon AL, Campbell JN, et al. Complications from silicon-polymer intubulation of nerves. Microsurgery 1989;10(2):130–3.
11. Dellon AL, Mackinnon SE. An alternative to the classical nerve graft for the management of the short nerve gap. Plast Reconstr Surg 1988;82(5):849–56.

12. Davis L, Perret G, Hiller F, et al. Experimental studies of peripheral nerve injuries. III. A study of recovery of function following repair by end to end sutures and nerve grafts. Surg Gyn Obst 1945;80:35–59.

13. Zalewski AA, Silvers WK. An evaluation of nerve repair with nerve allografts in normal and immunologically tolerant rats. J Neurosurg 1980;52(4): 557–63.

14. Levinthal R, Brown WJ, Rand RW. Fascicular nerve allograft evaluation. Part 2: comparison with whole-nerve allograft by light microscopy. J Neurosurg 1978;48(3):428–33.

15. Atchabahian A, Doolabh VB, Mackinnon SE, et al. Indefinite survival of peripheral nerve allografts after temporary Cyclosporine A immunosuppression. Restor Neurol Neurosci 1998;13(3–4):129–39.

16. Midha R, Evans PJ, Mackinnon SE, et al. Temporary immunosuppression for peripheral nerve allografts. Transplant Proc 1993;25(1 Pt 1):532–6.

17. Mackinnon SE, Hudson AR, Bain JR, et al. The peripheral nerve allograft: an assessment of regeneration in the immunosuppressed host. Plast Reconstr Surg 1987;79(3):436–46.

18. Midha R, Mackinnon SE, Becker LE. The fate of Schwann cells in peripheral nerve allografts. J Neuropathol Exp Neurol 1994;53(3):316–22.

19. Mackinnon SE, Doolabh VB, Novak CB, et al. Clinical outcome following nerve allograft transplantation. Plast Reconstr Surg 2001;107(6):1419–29.

20. Lundborg G. Nerve injury and repair: regeneration, reconstruction and cortical remodeling. Philadelphia: Elsevier; 2004.

21. Karabekmez FE, Duymaz A, Moran SL. Early clinical outcomes with the use of decellularized nerve allograft for repair of sensory defects within the hand. Hand (N Y) 2009;4(3):245–9.

22. Johnson PJ, Newton P, Hunter DA, et al. Nerve endoneurial microstructure facilitates uniform distribution of regenerative fibers: a post hoc comparison of midgraft nerve fiber densities. J Reconstr Microsurg 2011;27(2):83–90.

23. Isaacs J. Treatment of acute peripheral nerve injuries: current concepts. J Hand Surg Am 2010; 35(3):491–7 [quiz: 498].

24. Moore AM, MacEwan M, Santosa KB, et al. Acellular nerve allografts in peripheral nerve regeneration: a comparative study. Muscle Nerve 2011; 44(2):221–34.

25. Brooks DN, Weber RV, Chao JD, et al. Processed nerve allografts for peripheral nerve reconstruction: a multicenter study of utilization and outcomes in sensory, mixed, and motor nerve reconstructions. Microsurgery 2012;32(1):1–14.

26. Cho MS, Rinker BD, Weber RV, et al. Functional outcome following nerve repair in the upper extremity using processed nerve allograft. J Hand Surg Am 2012;37(11):2340–9.

27. Whitlock EL, Tuffaha SH, Luciano JP, et al. Processed allografts and type I collagen conduits for repair of peripheral nerve gaps. Muscle Nerve 2009;39(6):787–99.

28. Kerns JM, Danielsen N, Holmquist B, et al. The influence of predegeneration on regeneration through peripheral nerve grafts in the rat. Exp Neurol 1993;122(1):28–36.

29. Danielsen N, Kerns JM, Holmquist B, et al. Pre-degenerated nerve grafts enhance regeneration by shortening the initial delay period. Brain Res 1994;666(2):250–4.

30. Trumble TE. Peripheral nerve transplantation: the effects of predegenerated grafts and immunosuppression. J Neural Transplant Plast 1992;3(1):39–49.

31. Dubuisson AS, Foidart-Dessalle M, Reznik M, et al. Predegenerated nerve allografts versus fresh nerve allografts in nerve repair. Exp Neurol 1997; 148(1):378–87.

32. Lee HK, Chung MS, Kim HJ. A comparison of the passage of regenerating axons through old degenerated nerve autografts and fresh nerve autografts in rats. Int Orthop 1993;17(3):193–7.

33. George R, Griffin JW. Delayed macrophage responses and myelin clearance during Wallerian degeneration in the central nervous system: the dorsal radiculotomy model. Exp Neurol 1994; 129(2):225–36.

34. Lassner F, Becker M, Berger A. Degeneration and regeneration in nerve autografts and allografts. Microsurgery 1995;16(1):4–8.

35. Siironen J, Sandberg M, Vuorinen V, et al. Expression of type I and III collagens and fibronectin after transection of rat sciatic nerve. Reinnervation compared with denervation. Lab Invest 1992; 67(1):80–7.

36. Salonen V, Aho H, Roytta M, et al. Quantitation of Schwann cells and endoneurial fibroblast-like cells after experimental nerve trauma. Acta Neuropathol 1988;75(4):331–6.

37. Daniloff JK, Levi G, Grumet M, et al. Altered expression of neuronal cell adhesion molecules induced by nerve injury and repair. J Cell Biol 1986;103(3):929–45.

38. Meyer M, Matsuoka I, Wetmore C, et al. Enhanced synthesis of brain-derived neurotrophic factor in the lesioned peripheral nerve: different mechanisms are responsible for the regulation of BDNF and NGF mRNA. J Cell Biol 1992;119(1):45–54.

39. Kwok JC, Afshari F, Garcia-Alias G, et al. Proteoglycans in the central nervous system: plasticity, regeneration and their stimulation with chondroitinase ABC. Restor Neurol Neurosci 2008;26(2–3): 131–45.

40. Neubauer D, Graham JB, Muir D. Chondroitinase treatment increases the effective length of acellular nerve grafts. Exp Neurol 2007;207(1):163–70.

41. Zuo J, Hernandez YJ, Muir D. Chondroitin sulfate proteoglycan with neurite-inhibiting activity is up-regulated following peripheral nerve injury. J Neurobiol 1998;34(1):41–54.

42. Bungner OV. Degenerations-und regeneration-vorgänge am nerven nach verietzungen. Beitr Pathol Anat 1891;10:312–93.

43. Anderson PN, Turmaine M. Axonal regeneration through arterial grafts. J Anat 1986;147:73–82.

44. Weiss P, Taylor AC. Further experimental evidence against 'Neurotropism' in nerve regeneration. J Exp Zool 1944;95:233–57.

45. Kosutic D, Krajnc I, Pejkovic B, et al. Autogenous digital artery graft for repair of digital nerve defects in emergency hand reconstruction: two-year follow-up. J Plast Reconstr Aesthet Surg 2009;62(4):553.

46. Platt H. On the results of bridging gaps in injured nerve trunks by autogenous fascial tubulization and autogenous nerve grafts. Br J Surg 1919; 7(27):384–9.

47. Wrede L. Uberbruckung eines nervendefektes mittels seidennhat und lebenden venenstuckes. Dtsch Med Wochenschr 1909;35:1125.

48. Walton RL, Brown RE, Matory WE, et al. Autogenous vein graft repair of digital nerve defects in the finger: a retrospective clinical study. Plast Reconstr Surg 1989;84(6):944–9 [discussion: 950–2].

49. Chiu DT, Strauch B. A prospective clinical evaluation of autogenous vein grafts used as a nerve conduit for distal sensory nerve defects of 3 cm or less. Plast Reconstr Surg 1990;86(5):928–34.

50. Rinker B, Liau JY. A prospective randomized study comparing woven polyglycolic acid and autogenous vein conduits for reconstruction of digital nerve gaps. J Hand Surg Am 2011;36(5):775–81.

51. Wolford LM, Stevao EL. Considerations in nerve repair. Proc (Bayl Univ Med Cent) 2003;16(2): 152–6.

52. Edgar D, Timpl R, Thoenen H. The heparin-binding domain of laminin is responsible for its effects on neurite outgrowth and neuronal survival. EMBO J 1984;3(7):1463–8.

53. Lundborg G, Dahlin L, Danielsen N, et al. Trophism, tropism, and specificity in nerve regeneration. J Reconstr Microsurg 1994;10(5):345–54.

54. Tang JB. Group fascicular vein grafts with interposition of nerve slices for long ulnar nerve defects: report of three cases. Microsurgery 1993;14(6):404–8.

55. Tang JB. Vein conduits with interposition of nerve tissue for peripheral nerve defects. J Reconstr Microsurg 1995;11(1):21–6.

56. Brunelli GA, Battiston B, Vigasio A, et al. Bridging nerve defects with combined skeletal muscle and vein conduits. Microsurgery 1993;14(4):247–51.

57. Battiston B, Tos P, Cushway TR, et al. Nerve repair by means of vein filled with muscle grafts I. Clinical results. Microsurgery 2000;20(1):32–6.

58. Brooke R, Seckel MD, Jones D, et al. Hyaluronic acid through a new injectable nerve guide delivery system enhances peripheral nerve regeneration in the rat. J Neurosci Res 2004;40(3): 318–24.

59. Nishiura Y, Brandt J, Nilsson A, et al. Addition of cultured Schwann cells to tendon autografts and freeze-thawed muscle grafts improves peripheral nerve regeneration. Tissue Eng 2004;10(1–2): 157–64.

60. Brandt J, Dahlin LB, Lundborg G. Autologous tendons used as grafts for bridging peripheral nerve defects. J Hand Surg Br 1999;24(3):284–90.

61. Luo YX, Chao DC. An experimental study of using "tendon bridge" or "tendon tunnel" as a conduit for nerve regeneration. J Tongji Med Univ 1989; 9(2):103–6.

62. Brandt J, Dahlin LB, Kanje M, et al. Functional recovery in a tendon autograft used to bridge a peripheral nerve defect. Scand J Plast Reconstr Surg Hand Surg 2002;36(1):2–8.

63. Lundborg G, Rosen B, Dahlin L, et al. Tubular versus conventional repair of median and ulnar nerves in the human forearm: early results from a prospective, randomized, clinical study. J Hand Surg Am 1997;22(1):99–106.

64. Lundborg G, Rosen B, Abrahamson SO, et al. Tubular repair of the median nerve in the human forearm. Preliminary findings. J Hand Surg Br 1994;19(3):273–6.

65. Lundborg G, Dahlin LB, Danielsen N. Ulnar nerve repair by the silicone chamber technique. Case report. Scand J Plast Reconstr Surg Hand Surg 1991;25(1):79–82.

66. Moore AM, Kasukurthi R, Magill CK, et al. Limitations of conduits in peripheral nerve repairs. Hand (N Y) 2009;4(2):180–6.

67. Rosson GD, Williams EH, Dellon AL. Motor nerve regeneration across a conduit. Microsurgery 2009;29(2):107–14.

68. Mackinnon SE, Dellon AL. Clinical nerve reconstruction with a bioabsorbable polyglycolic acid tube. Plast Reconstr Surg 1990;85(3):419–24.

69. Weber RA, Breidenbach WC, Brown RE, et al. A randomized prospective study of polyglycolic acid conduits for digital nerve reconstruction in humans. Plast Reconstr Surg 2000;106(5): 1036–45 [discussion: 1046–8].

70. Battiston B, Tos P, Cushway TR, et al. Nerve repair by means of tubulization: literature review and personal clinical experience comparing biological and synthetic conduits for sensory nerve repair. Microsurgery 2005;25(4):258–67.

71. Bushnell BD, McWilliams AD, Whitener GB, et al. Early clinical experience with collagen nerve tubes in digital nerve repair. J Hand Surg Am 2008;33(7): 1081–7.

72. Wangensteen KJ, Kalliainen LK. Collagen tube conduits in peripheral nerve repair: a retrospective analysis. Hand (N Y) 2010;5(3):273–7.

73. Lohmeyer JA, Siemers F, Machens HG, et al. The clinical use of artificial nerve conduits for digital nerve repair: a prospective cohort study and literature review. J Reconstr Microsurg 2009;25(1):55–61.

74. Thomsen L, Bellemere P, Loubersac T, et al. Treatment by collagen conduit of painful post-traumatic neuromas of the sensitive digital nerve: a retrospective study of 10 cases. Chir Main 2010;29(4):255–62.

75. Taras JS, Jacoby SM, Lincoski CJ. Reconstruction of digital nerves with collagen conduits. J Hand Surg Am 2011;36(9):1441–6.

76. Bertleff MJ, Meek MF, Nicolai JP. A prospective clinical evaluation of biodegradable neurolac nerve guides for sensory nerve repair in the hand. J Hand Surg Am 2005;30(3):513–8.

77. Meek MF, Nicolai JP, Robinson PH. Secondary digital nerve repair in the foot with resorbable p(DLLA-epsilon-CL) nerve conduits. J Reconstr Microsurg 2006;22(3):149–51.

78. Hernandez-Cortes P, Garrido J, Camara M, et al. Failed digital nerve reconstruction by foreign body reaction to Neurolac nerve conduit. Microsurgery 2010;30:414–6.

79. Chiriac S, Facca S, Diaconu M, et al. Experience of using the bioresorbable copolyester poly(DL-lactide-epsilon-caprolactone) nerve conduit guide Neurolac for nerve repair in peripheral nerve defects: report on a series of 28 lesions. J Hand Surg Eur Vol 2012;37(4):342–9.

80. Hall H. Modified fibrin hydrogel matrices: both, 3D-scaffolds and local and controlled release systems to stimulate angiogenesis. Curr Pharm Des 2007;13(35):3597–607.

81. Sameem M, Wood TJ, Bain JR. A systematic review on the use of fibrin glue for peripheral nerve repair. Plast Reconstr Surg 2011;127(6):2381–90.

82. Kalbermatten DF, Pettersson J, Kingham PJ, et al. New fibrin conduit for peripheral nerve repair. J Reconstr Microsurg 2009;25(1):27–33.

83. Pettersson J, Kalbermatten D, McGrath A, et al. Biodegradable fibrin conduit promotes long-term regeneration after peripheral nerve injury in adult rats. J Plast Reconstr Aesthet Surg 2010;63(11):1893–9.

84. Temple CL, Ross DC, Dunning CE, et al. Resistance to disruption and gapping of peripheral nerve repairs: an in vitro biomechanical assessment of techniques. J Reconstr Microsurg 2004;20(8):645–50.

85. Nishimura MT, Mazzer N, Barbieri CH, et al. Mechanical resistance of peripheral nerve repair with biological glue and with conventional suture at different postoperative times. J Reconstr Microsurg 2008;24(5):327–32.

86. Cruz NI, Debs N, Fiol RE. Evaluation of fibrin glue in rat sciatic nerve repairs. Plast Reconstr Surg 1986;78(3):369–73.

87. McGrath AM, Brohlin M, Kingham PJ, et al. Fibrin conduit supplemented with human mesenchymal stem cells and immunosuppressive treatment enhances regeneration after peripheral nerve injury. Neurosci Lett 2012;516(2):171–6.

88. Rafijah G, Bowen AJ, Dolores C, et al. The effects of adjuvant fibrin sealant on the surgical repair of segmental nerve defects. J Hand Surg Am 2013;38(5):847–55.

89. el-Barrany WG, Marei AG, Vallee B. Anatomic basis of vascularised nerve grafts: the blood supply of peripheral nerves. Surg Radiol Anat 1999;21(2):95–102.

90. Shibata M, Tsai TM, Firrell J, et al. Experimental comparison of vascularized and nonvascularized nerve grafting. J Hand Surg Am 1988;13(3):358–65.

91. Settergren CR, Wood MB. Comparison of blood flow in free vascularized versus nonvascularized nerve grafts. J Reconstr Microsurg 1984;1(2):95–101.

92. Daly PJ, Wood MB. Endoneural and epineural blood flow evaluation with free vascularized and conventional nerve grafts in the canine. J Reconstr Microsurg 1985;2(1):45–9.

93. Koshima I, Harii K. Experimental study of vascularized nerve grafts: morphometric study of axonal regeneration of nerves transplanted into silicone tubes. Ann Plast Surg 1985;14(3):235–43.

94. Lux P, Breidenbach W, Firrell J. Determination of temporal changes in blood flow in vascularized and nonvascularized nerve grafts in the dog. Plast Reconstr Surg 1988;82(1):133–44.

95. Tark KC, Roh TS. Morphometric study of regeneration through vascularized nerve graft in a rabbit sciatic nerve model. J Reconstr Microsurg 2001;17(2):109–14.

96. Saray A, Teoman Tellioglu A, Altinok G. Prefabrication of a free peripheral nerve graft following implantation on an arteriovenous pedicle. J Reconstr Microsurg 2002;18(4):281–8.

97. Serel S, Kaya B, Sara Y, et al. Is it possible to prefabricate a vascularized peripheral nerve graft? Ann Plast Surg 2010;64(3):323–6.

98. Kemp SW, Syed S, Walsh W, et al. Collagen nerve conduits promote enhanced axonal regeneration, schwann cell association, and neovascularization compared to silicone conduits. Tissue Eng Part A 2009;15(8):1975–88.

99. Hobson MI. Increased vascularisation enhances axonal regeneration within an acellular nerve conduit. Ann R Coll Surg Engl 2002;84(1):47–53.

100. Zheng L, Cui HF. Use of chitosan conduit combined with bone marrow mesenchymal stem cells for

promoting peripheral nerve regeneration. J Mater Sci Mater Med 2010;21(5):1713–20.

101. Gu J, Hu W, Deng A, et al. Surgical repair of a 30 mm long human median nerve defect in the distal forearm by implantation of a chitosan-PGA nerve guidance conduit. J Tissue Eng Regen Med 2012;6(2):163–8.

102. Guénard V, Kleitman N, Morrissey TK, et al. Syngenic Schwann cells derived from adult nerves seeded in semipermeable guidance channels enhance peripheral nerve regeneration. J Neurosci 1992;2:3310.

103. Santiago LY, Clavijo-Alvarez J, Brayfield C, et al. Delivery of adipose-derived precursor cells for peripheral nerve repair. Cell Transplant 2009;18(2):145–58.

104. Kalbermatten DF, Kingham PJ, Mahay D, et al. Fibrin matrix for suspension of regenerative cells in an artificial nerve conduit. J Plast Reconstr Aesthet Surg 2008;61(6):669–75.

105. Di Summa PG, Kingham PJ, Raffoul W, et al. Adipose-derived stem cells enhance peripheral nerve regeneration. J Plast Reconstr Aesthet Surg 2010;63:1544–52.

106. Chang CJ, Hsu SH. The effects of low-intensity ultrasound on peripheral nerve regeneration in poly(DL-lactic acid-co-glycolic acid) conduits seeded with Schwann cells. Ultrasound Med Biol 2004;30(8):1079–84.

107. Hadlock T, Sundback C, Hunter D, et al. A polymer foam conduit seeded with Schwann cells promotes guided peripheral nerve regeneration. Tissue Eng 2000;6(2):119–27.

108. Berrocal YA, Almeida VW, Gupta R, et al. Transplantation of Schwann cells within a collagen tube for the repair of large segmental peripheral nerve defects in rats. J Neurosurg, in press.

109. Oliveira JT, Almeida FM, Biancalana A, et al. Mesenchymal stem cells in a polycaprolactone conduit enhance median-nerve regeneration, prevent decrease of creatine phosphokinase levels in muscle, and improve functional recovery in mice. Neuroscience 2010;170(4):1295–303.

110. Liu BS, Yang YC, Shen CC. Regenerative effect of adipose tissue-derived stem cells transplantation using nerve conduit therapy on sciatic nerve injury in rats. J Tissue Eng Regen Med 2012. [Epub ahead of print].

111. McLeod M, Hong M, Mukhida K, et al. Erythropoietin and GDNF enhance ventral mesencephalic fiber outgrowth and capillary proliferation following neural transplantation in a rodent model of Parkinson's disease. Eur J Neurosci 2006;24(2):361–70.

112. Huang AH, Synder BR, Cheng PH, et al. Putative dental pulp-derived stem/stromal cells promote proliferation and differentiation of endogenous

neural cells in the hippocampus of mice. Stem Cells 2008;26(10):2654–63.

113. Arthur A, Rychkov G, Shi S, et al. Adult human dental pulp stem cells differentiate toward functionally active neurons under appropriate environmental cues. Stem Cells 2008;26(7):1787–95.

114. Xu Y, Liu L, Zhao C, et al. Neurospheres from rat adipose-derived stem cells could be induced into functional Schwann cell-like cells in vitro. BMC Neurosci 2008;9:21.

115. Fujimura J, Ogawa R, Mizuno H, et al. Neural differentiation of adipose-derived stem cells isolated from GFP transgenic mice. Biochem Biophys Res Commun 2005;333(1):116–21.

116. Zavan B, Vindigni V, Gardin C, et al. Neural potential of adipose stem cells. Discov Med 2010;10(50):37–43.

117. Rehman J, Traktuev D, Li J, et al. Secretion of angiogenic and antiapoptotic factors by human adipose stromal cells. Circulation 2004;109(10):1292–8.

118. Nosrat IV, Smith CA, Mullally P, et al. Dental pulp cells provide neurotrophic support for dopaminergic neurons and differentiate into neurons in vitro; implications for tissue engineering and repair in the nervous system. Eur J Neurosci 2004;19(9):2388–98.

119. Dai LG, Huang GS, Hsu SH. Sciatic nerve regeneration by co-cultured Schwann cells and stem cells on microporous nerve conduits. Cell Transplant 2012. [Epub ahead of print].

120. Yin Q, Kemp GJ, Yu LG, et al. Neurotrophin-4 delivered by fibrin glue promotes peripheral nerve regeneration. Muscle Nerve 2001;24(3):345–51.

121. Jubran M, Widenfalk J. Repair of peripheral nerve transections with fibrin sealant containing neurotrophic factors. Exp Neurol 2003;181(2):204–12.

122. Ehrbar M, Zeisberger SM, Raeber GP, et al. The role of actively released fibrin-conjugated VEGF for VEGF receptor 2 gene activation and the enhancement of angiogenesis. Biomaterials 2008;29(11):1720–9.

123. Fine EG, Decosterd I, Papaloizos M, et al. GDNF and NGF released by synthetic guidance channels support sciatic nerve regeneration across a long gap. Eur J Neurosci 2002;15(4):589–601.

124. Madduri S, Feldman K, Tervoort T, et al. Collagen nerve conduits releasing the neurotrophic factors GDNF and NGF. J Control Release 2010;143(2):168–74.

125. Moore AM, Wood MD, Chenard K, et al. Controlled delivery of glial cell line-derived neurotrophic factor enhances motor nerve regeneration. J Hand Surg Am 2010;35(12):2008–17.

126. Wood MD, MacEwan MR, French AR, et al. Fibrin matrices with affinity-based delivery systems and neurotrophic factors promote functional nerve regeneration. Biotechnol Bioeng 2010;106(6):970–9.

127. Xie J, Li X, Xia Y. Putting electrospun nanofibers to work for biomedical research. Macromol Rapid Commun 2008;29(22):1775–92.

128. Jin J, Park M, Rengarajan A, et al. Functional motor recovery after peripheral nerve repair with an aligned nanofiber tubular conduit in a rat model. Regen Med 2012;7(6):799–806.

129. Zhan X, Gao M, Jiang Y, et al. Nanofiber scaffolds facilitate functional regeneration of peripheral nerve injury. Nanomedicine 2012;9(3):305–15.

130. Hu X, Huang J, Ye Z, et al. A novel scaffold with longitudinally oriented microchannels promotes peripheral nerve regeneration. Tissue Eng Part A 2009;15(11):3297–308.

131. Roy J, Kennedy TE, Costantino S. Engineered cell culture substrates for axon guidance studies: moving beyond proof of concept. Lab Chip 2013; 13(4):498–508.

132. Dudanova I, Klein R. Integration of guidance cues: parallel signaling and crosstalk. Trends Neurosci 2013;36(5):295–304.

133. Donoghoe N, Rosson GD, Dellon AL. Reconstruction of the human median nerve in the forearm with the Neurotube. Microsurgery 2007;27(7): 595–600.

134. Dellon AL, Maloney CT Jr. Salvage of sensation in a hallux-to-thumb transfer by nerve tube reconstruction. J Hand Surg Am 2006;31(9):1495–8.

How to Measure Outcomes of Peripheral Nerve Surgery

Yirong Wang, MD[a], Malay Sunitha, MPH[b],
Kevin C. Chung, MD, MS[c],*

KEYWORDS

- Peripheral nerve • Hand surgery • Outcomes assessment

KEY POINTS

- Outcomes assessment tools and the current choices of measurements in outcomes research of peripheral nerve surgery.
- Several aspects relating to function, pain, and patient perception of outcomes are evaluated after peripheral nerve repair.
- Choice of specific measures depends on the researcher's interest and the disease or treatment under investigation.

The outcomes movement, initiated in 1988, was stimulated by the national emphasis on cost containment and efforts to limit geographic differences in the use of various medical procedures.[1–3] Goals of the outcomes movement included "increased understanding of the effectiveness of different interventions, the use of this information to make possible better decision making by physicians and patients, and the development of standards to guide physicians and aid third-party payers in optimizing the use of resources, by investigating and comparing patient experiences."[1,4] Patient experiences can range from mortality, physiologic measures, reduction of symptoms, improvement in daily functioning, and clinical events to patient satisfaction.[4,5] The outcomes chosen to evaluate care need to be carefully considered based on criteria that are most pertinent to the patient's need. Additionally vital are the criteria for selecting outcome measurement instruments, which comprise reliability, validity, and responsiveness of measures, their clinical usefulness, and relationship to the care under investigation.[5]

Peripheral nerve injuries can be caused by trauma, accidental injuries during extensive surgery, nerve tumors, compressive disease, or congenital anomalies, with most (81%) located on an upper extremity.[6,7] Among upper-limb or lower-limb trauma, incidence of nerve injuries is reported to be 1.64%, with crush injuries having the highest rate, at 1.9%.[8] These injuries may lead to irreversible disabilities in patients, such as sensory loss, deficient motor function, pain problems in terms of cold intolerance and hyperesthesia, which impair hand function and affect quality of life at work and in society.[7] Despite marked advances in neuroscience, peripheral nerve injuries continue to pose challenges for surgical reconstruction, because the clinical outcomes still seem unsatisfactory.[6,7] Advances in this field require accurate measures of treatment

Supported in part by a Midcareer Investigator Award in Patient-Oriented Research (K24 AR053120) from the National Institute of Arthritis and Musculoskeletal and Skin Diseases (to Dr Kevin C. Chung).
[a] 17th Department of Plastic Surgery, Plastic Surgery Hospital, Peking Union Medical College, Chinese Academy of Medical Science, 33 Ba-Da-Chu Road, Beijing 100144, China; [b] Section of Plastic Surgery, Department of Surgery, University of Michigan Health System, East Medical Center Drive, Ann Arbor, MI 48109, USA; [c] Section of Plastic Surgery, University of Michigan Medical School, University of Michigan Health System, 2130 Taubman Center, SPC 5340, 1500 East Medical Center Drive, Ann Arbor, MI 48109-5340, USA
* Corresponding author.
E-mail address: kecchung@umich.edu

effectiveness to assess new treatments, which are forthcoming.

The assessment of recovery after peripheral nerve surgery remains a challenging process to therapists and surgeons. Numerous cellular and biochemical mechanisms that occur in peripheral and central nervous systems affect the outcomes and result in difficult evaluation of recovery.[9] Measurement instruments for peripheral nerve surgery need to aid clinical diagnosis, assess and compare surgical repair techniques, track rehabilitation progress, provide feedback to both patient and therapist, as well as ascertain disability after injury.[9] The list of objectives useful in evaluation of hand function after peripheral nerve repair is provided in **Table 1**. Outcomes research after nerve injury has recently had an emphasis more on functional results and patient-reported outcomes.[10–13] This review focuses on the scope of outcomes assessment tools and the current choices of measurements in outcomes research of peripheral nerve surgery. **Table 2** details available methods for assessing patient outcomes after peripheral nerve surgeries.

OUTCOMES ASSESSMENT

Outcomes assessment in peripheral nerve injuries can be broadly categorized into tests of sensory function, motor function, pain and discomfort, and neurophysiologic and patient-reported outcomes.

Sensory Function

Sensory tests indicate the sensory acuity of the hand and how well the patient is able to use it.[14] The Semmes-Weinstein monofilament test is used to assess perception of cutaneous pressure threshold, which reflects reinnervation of peripheral targets.[15] Compared with using a common tuning fork, the test provides quantitative data, which can be used to follow a patient serially during the course of nerve regeneration.[16] Tactile gnosis is the capability of the hand to recognize the character of objects, such as shapes and textures, and is a prime marker of functional recovery.[17] Two-point discrimination (2PD) is an established assessment tool for tactile gnosis.[17] The static 2PD test (S2PD) measures the innervation density of the slowly adapting receptor (which fires continuously if pressure is applied) population.[14] One study showed an age-related decline in the ability to discriminate 2 points, and there was no significant difference between men and women.[18] The moving 2PD test (M2PD) relies on the quickly adapting receptor system (which fires at onset and offset of stimulation), which recovers sooner and in larger numbers.[19] The threshold values are lower than those of the static test.[20] However, 2PD outcome in nerve repair studies is reported to be variable, because there is a lack of standardization of the technique and the test is probably performed in different ways by different investigators.[21] It is a serious problem because the test is frequently used to compare different nerve repair techniques. Therefore, when 2PD results are reported in a study, a detailed and referenced description, especially the pressure applied and the testing protocol, should be mandatory.[21] Dellon[22] has introduced a pressure-specifying sensory device to provide a standardized pressure; however, it may be difficult to use this technique in routine clinical practice. The 2PD test is not recommended as the only instrument to monitor sensory function. Localization of touch and identification based on active touching are also recommended to be assessed for an overall evaluation of sensory function.[21] Other functional sensory tests include shape, texture identification,[23,24] vibration, and

Table 1
List of objectives to evaluate hand function after peripheral nerve repair

	Name of the Objective	Objective
1	Reinnervation	To demonstrate regeneration of the nerve and reinnervation of muscles and cutaneous receptors
2	Tactile gnosis	To determine the ability to interpret the new sensory input
3	Dexterity, grip strength, and activities of daily living capacity	To assess skills requiring integrated sensory and motor functions of the hand
4	Pain, discomfort	To quantify the degree of pain and discomfort in terms of hypersensitivity and cold intolerance

Data from Rosen B. Recovery of sensory and motor function after nerve repair. A rationale for evaluation. J Hand Ther 1996;9:315–27; with permission.

Table 2
Outcomes assessment tools for measuring outcomes after peripheral nerve surgeries

Measurement	Characteristics							
Sensory Function								
S2PD[14,18]	The minimal distance at which 2 points can be discriminated is measured. The 2 points of a caliper are applied at the same time using the weight of the caliper alone ("Just blanching the skin"[21])	Normal values (age, y)						
			10-19	20-29	30-39	40-49	50-59	60-69	70-79
		Men (mm) (mean ± standard deviation)	6.1 ± 2.7	6.7 ± 2.5	7.2 ± 3.6	7.9 ± 2.6	8.8 ± 4.9	9.3 ± 3.8	9.1 ± 2.7
		Women (mean ± standard deviation)	6.5 ± 2.5	7.5 ± 4.0	7.6 ± 3.1	8.1 ± 3.1	9.0 ± 3.4	9.3 ± 3.7	10.9 ± 4.8
		American Society for Surgery of the Hand classification[71]: <6 mm is normal, 6–10 mm is fair, and 11–15 mm is poor							
M2PD[14,19]	Performed by moving the calipers over the skin surface	The threshold values are lower than those of the static test							
Area localization[14,24]	The territory of the injured nerve is divided into different zones, with the hand hidden from patient's sight. Patients are tested on their ability to localize a light touch applied to each zone in random order								
Pick-up test[29]	Patients are required to pick up small objects and place them in a container with and without vision								
British MRC Score of sensory recovery modified by Mackinnon and Dellon[23,28,72]	S0: absence of sensibility in the autonomous area of the nerve S1: recovery of deep cutaneous pain and tactile sensibility S1+: recovery of superficial pain sensibility S2: recovery of some degree of superficial cutaneous pain and tactile sensibility S2+: as in S2, but with overresponse S3: return of pain and tactile sensibility with disappearance of overresponse; S2PD >15 mm, M2PD >7 mm S3+: return of sensibility as in S3 with some recovery of 2-point discrimination; S2PD: 7–15 mm, M2PD: 4–7 mm S4: complete recovery; S2PD: 2–6 mm, M2PD: 2–3 mm								
Semmes-Weinstein monofilament test[9]	Used to evaluate cutaneous pressure thresholds. Detection threshold defined as perceived sensation after application of the smallest Semmes-Weinstein monofilament at the affected fingertip 0 = untestable 1 (filament marking 6.65) = perception of deep pressure 2 (filament marking 4.56) = loss of protective sensation 3 (filament marking 4.31) = diminished protective sensation 4 (filament marking 3.61) = diminished perception of light touch 5 (filament marking 2.83) = normal perception of touch and pressure								

(continued on next page)

Table 2
(continued)

Measurement	Characteristics		
Vibration perception[26]	Evaluated with tuning forks		
Temperature perception[25,26]	Test ability to discriminate warm and cold objects		
Recognition of textures[23,24,26]	Differentiation between different textures, with the patient wearing protective earmuffs to eliminate auditory input		
Recognition of shape[24,26]	Differentiation between small, easily manipulated, three-dimensional shapes		
Sharp and dull discrimination[25]	Test ability to discriminate sharp and dull stimuli		
Thickness discrimination[26]	Differentiation between blocks 1-cm, 2-cm, and 3-cm thick		
Finger Dexterity			
Sollerman hand function test[23]	Consists of 20 tasks based on the most common hand grips		
Motor Function			
MMT[31]	Conducted to assess motor innervation using MRC muscle strength grading system.		
British MRC muscle strength grading system[73]	M0: no contraction		
	M1: flicker or trace of contraction		
	M2: full range of active movement, with gravity eliminated		
	M3: active movement against gravity		
	M4: active movement against gravity and resistance		
	M5: normal power		
Modified MRC muscle strength scale[31]	Grade	Range of movement	Resistance
	0	None	No palpable contraction
	1	None	Palpable contraction only
	2	Reduced	None
	3	Normal	None
	4	Normal	Reduced
	5	Normal	Normal

Grip strength[4,32]	Measured with a dynamometer. The result from the noninjured hand is considered normal. Can measure standard dynamic grip strength; time to achieve 95% of maximum grip strength; maximum power outputs
Pinch strength[32]	Key (lateral) pinch: influenced by thumb interphalangeal joint position, first dorsal IOM, flexor pollicis longus, flexor pollicis brevis Tip to tip (thumb pulp to index pulp) pinch and tripod (thumb pulp to index and middle finger pulps) pinch: rely on thenar muscles
Pain and Discomfort	
Numerical Rating Scale for pain[59,74,75]	Consists of asking the patient to rate their perceived level of pain intensity on a numerical scale from 0 to 100, with the 0 representing "no pain" and 100 representing "pain as bad as it could be"
Pain Visual Analogue Scale[11,54,76,77]	Consists of a 10-cm line anchored by 2 extremes of pain, including "no pain" and "pain as bad as it could be." The scale is scored by measuring the distance from the beginning to the patient's mark
Pain Disability Index[33]	7-item questionnaire designed to assess the extent to which pain interferes with daily life domains
McGill Pain Questionnaire[35,77]	Designed to provide quantitative measures of clinical pain
McCabe Cold Sensitivity Severity Scale[39,77,78]	Consists of 4 questions about events in the home that cause cold-related symptoms. Patients are asked to mark on a 10-cm line to reflect the severity of cold intolerance during the activities. The score is summed by measuring the distance from the beginning to the patient's mark of each question
McCabe Potential Work-Exposure Scale[39]	Consists of 3 questions about exposure of the hands to cold in the workplace. Patients are asked to mark on a 10-cm line to reflect the severity of cold intolerance during the activities. The scale is scored by measuring the distance from the beginning to the mark, and then summing the score
Cold Intolerance Symptom Severity questionnaire[77]	Consists of 6 questions that highlight the impact of cold intolerance on daily life. The first question concerns pattern of cold intolerance and severity of symptoms, which is not included in the final score

(continued on next page)

Table 2
(continued)

Measurement	Characteristics
Electroneurophysiologic Outcomes Measures	
Electroneurography examinations[51]	Include sensory and motor nerve measurements, such as SCVs and amplitude, MCVs, distal motor latency
Electromyogram examinations[53]	Used to test muscle innervation
Grading scales for neurophysiological changes of median nerve entrapment classified by Bland[48]	Grade 0 — Normal
	Grade 1 — (Very mild) CTS shown only with most sensitive tests
	Grade 2 — (Mild) SCVs slow on finger/wrist measurement, normal terminal motor latency
	Grade 3 — (Moderate) distal motor latency to APB <6.5 ms with preserved sensory nerve action potential
	Grade 4 — (Severe) absent sensory nerve action potential but motor response preserved, and distal motor latency to APB <6.5 ms
	Grade 5 — (Very severe) motor terminal latency >6.5 ms
	Grade 6 — (Extremely severe) sensory and motor potentials effectively unrecordable (surface motor potential from APB <0.2 mV amplitude)

Overall Hand Function Classification for Ulnar Nerve Injury

Akahori's classification for staging of ulnar nerve injury preoperative status[51]

	Nerve conduction velocity		Clinical signs			
				Motor nerve		
	Motor nerve	Sensory nerve	Sensory nerve	Muscle atrophy	Motor weakness	Finger deformity
Stage I	Normal	Normal	Elbow flexion test (+) Hypesthesia (slightly +)	Only in first dorsal interosseous muscle (first IOM) (+ or −)	+ or −	−
Stage II	Normal	Delayed	Hypesthesia (+) commonly preceded by hypalgesia	First IOM (+) Other muscles (+ or −)	+ or −	+ or −
Stage III	Lower limit or delayed	Delayed or immeasurable	Hypesthesia (+)	+	+	+
Stage IV	Delayed	Immeasurable	Hypesthesia (2+), sometimes analgesia	2+	2+	2+
Stage V	Delayed or immeasurable	Immeasurable	Hypesthesia (2+), mostly analgesia	2+	2+	2+

Akahori's criteria for measuring ulnar nerve functional recovery[51]	Excellent	Normal; no motor weakness, can include slight muscle atrophy, coldness in fingers, subtle hypesthesia
	Good	Muscle strength rated 4 or 5 in MMT, no residual deformity, some hypesthesia that does not impair ADLs
	Fair	Clinical improvement, but the claw finger deformity, disability of small finger adduction, and Froment sign may remain; hypesthesia that impairs ADLs
	Poor	No improvement or worsening
McGowan's classification for ulnar nerve injury[79]	Grade I	Minimal lesions, with no detectable motor weakness of the hand
	Grade II	Intermediate lesions
	Grade III	Severe lesions, with paralysis of ≥1 of the ulnar intrinsic muscles
Patient-Reported Outcomes		
Disability of the Arm, Shoulder, and Hand questionnaires[10,59,73]		30-item questionnaire that addresses arm-specific symptoms and disability during the preceding week. Used to estimate the patient's view of disability
Boston Carpal Tunnel Questionnaire[47,66]		Include symptom severity score and function score, assess severity of symptoms and functional status in patients who have CTS
Michigan Hand Outcomes Questionnaire[56]		37-item questionnaire assess disability along 6 domains: function, ADLs, pain, hand appearance, patient satisfaction, and work disability
Short Form-36[10]		General health assessment questionnaire, assess patient's quality of life, including 8 domains

Abbreviations: +, positive; −, negative; ADL, activities of daily living; APB, abductor pollicis brevis; CTS, carpal tunnel syndrome; IOM, interosseous muscle; M2PD, moving 2-point discrimination test; MCVs, motor nerve conduction velocities; MMT, manual muscle testing; MRC, Medical Research Council; S2PD, static 2-point discrimination test; SCVs, sensory nerve conduction velocities.

temperature perception, sharp and dull discrimination, and thickness discrimination.[25,26] These tests are timed and the results are converted into scores in multiple ways.[23–26]

The Medical Research Council (MRC) Scale, published in 1954,[27] is commonly used, by including 2PD for grading the sensory outcome after peripheral nerve surgery.[17,23,28] This scale is categorized into S0 to S4: S0 is the absence of sensibility; S1 is the recovery of deep cutaneous pain; S2 is the return of superficial cutaneous pain and some degree of tactile sensibility; S3 is the return of superficial cutaneous pain and tactile sensibility without overresponse; and S4 is complete recovery.[23] This scale has also been criticized because it is based on subjective findings and vague nonstandardized data. It is recommended to be used with additional evaluation of motor recovery and pain.[23] Moberg proposed the pick-up test as an objective method to measure integrated function of the hand by scoring both the speed and accuracy of identification of the test objects.[24,29]

Finger Dexterity

The Sollerman hand function test consists of 20 activities that replicate the main hand grips in daily living and is used to evaluate the quality of basic grip types.[30] Each subtest is scored depending on the quality of the hand grip and the patient's difficulty in performing the task.[9] This test can reflect integrated sensory and motor functions.[9]

Motor Function

Manual muscle testing is used to assess motor innervation using British Medical Research Council muscle strength grading.[31] It can be conducted to assess larger muscles or muscle groups, as well as intrinsic muscles of the hand. For the median nerve, palmar abduction in the thumb is evaluated. For the ulnar nerve, abduction in index and small finger and adduction in small finger are tested.[23,31] Brandsma[31] made some modifications to the MRC grades definitions, which were defined by range of motion and resistance, and made it more practical for intrinsic muscles of the hand. Assessment of grip strength with dynamometry is a most common method of reporting motor outcome.[32] Power grip requires synergistic function of intrinsic and extrinsic muscles of the hand, so it is difficult to determine muscle dysfunction in isolation with this test.[4] It is also influenced by pain or increased sensitivity to pressure over the pillar region or scar, and should not be used when tissue healing is incomplete and testing would cause pain.[32] Pinch strength tests include key pinch, tip pinch, and

tripod pinch. Tip pinch and tripod pinch dynamometry more specifically target the thenar musculature and seem to be more responsive for assessing motor function after carpal tunnel release, compared with grip and key pinch strength test.[32]

Pain and Discomfort

Pain is associated with disability in patients after peripheral nerve injury.[33] The evaluation of pain is always a self-report by patients. Numerical Rating Scale (NRS) for pain and Pain Visual Analogue Scale (PVAS) are used to determine pain intensity and are easy to use. However, there are some deficiencies about these measurements.[34] First, they assume that pain is a linear continuous phenomenon, which is not tenable in most cases. Second, all patients cannot respond to these scales in a uniform manner, because of the high variability in the pain they experience.[34] McGill Pain Questionnaire is a multidimensional pain scale, which provides more information on dimensions of pain beyond the simple factor of intensity, such as sensory components (tingling and hypersensitivity) as well as affective responses to pain.[33–36] However, it is a long questionnaire and imposes a larger burden on patients and might be less responsive than PVAS.[34] The Pain Disability Index assesses the impact of pain on life domains.[33] It includes 7 categories of life activity: family/home responsibility, recreation, social activity, occupation, sexual behavior, self-care, and life support activity.[37] Consistency, validity and reliability of this questionnaire were tested and proved to be useful in nerve injury studies.[33] In patients with chronic nerve injury, pain intensity is only 1 component of pain, and the impact of pain in the disability should also be considered.[33] A clear understanding of the goal of the research question helps determine which measurement is appropriate.

Cold sensitivity is a complex symptom, which may present as pain, numbness, stiffness, weakness, swelling, and change in skin color. The Cold Sensitivity Severity (CSS) Scale is used to evaluate sensitivity of cold intolerance during daily life.[38] The Potential Work-Exposure Scale assesses exposure in the work place.[38] The CSS Scale, in conjunction with the Potential Work-Exposure Scale, can be used to predict the likelihood of the patient's return to preinjury employment.[39] The reliability and validity of these 2 questionnaires have been shown in the development phase and in other studies.[38,39] The Cold Intolerance Symptom Severity questionnaire is a reliable and valid measurement, with a threshold value for pathologic cold intolerance of 30[40] and 50 for a population in a Scandinavian climate.[41]

Neurophysiologic Outcome Measurements

Neurophysiologic examinations include electro-neurography (ENG), also known as nerve conduction studies (including sensory nerve conduction velocity and amplitude, motor nerve velocity, distal motor latency), and electromyography (EMG). They measure the electrical activity of muscles and nerves and are the primary studies used to gain information on the location, number, and pathophysiology of lesions affecting the peripheral nerve.[42] In evaluation of carpal tunnel syndrome (CTS), distal motor latency, and sensory nerve conduction velocity are often performed. The American Association of Electrodiagnostic Medicine, American Academy of Neurology, and American Academy of Physical Medicine and Rehabilitation published the parameters for performing CTS electrodiagnostic testing to address the best electrodiagnostic studies to confirm the diagnosis and guide clinical researches.[43] Studies of ENG in patients with CTS have presented contradictory results among neurophysiologic findings, patient symptoms, and clinical improvements.[44–47] However, these studies did not refute the necessity of conducting ENG when evaluating patients with CTS.[44–47] Grading scales for the neurophysiologic changes of median nerve entrapment were also introduced to facilitate comparison of the severity of the disease.[47,48] A study showed that both ENG and patient-oriented questionnaires were highly responsive to treatment of CTS, but no correlation was observed between them. Therefore both outcome measurements are recommended to provide a multifaceted assessment.[49] ENG test can also be used to evaluate outcomes of nerve grafting,[50] nerve repair,[25] and cubital tunnel syndrome.[51,52] Patients showed continued improvement in sensory and motor nerve conduction velocity even beyond 2 years in cubital tunnel syndrome.[51] In brachial plexus injury, EMG is commonly used to evaluate muscle reinnervation.[53]

Patient-Reported Outcomes

There is a shift toward using patient-reported outcome with valid and reliable measurement tools in hand surgery. In a systematic review of studies of outcomes of hand surgery, quality-of-life outcomes were reported in 31% of the studies, comprising symptoms, patient satisfaction, and time to return to work and data from questionnaires related to quality of life.[2] Questionnaires commonly used in peripheral nerve surgery

outcome studies include Short Form 36 (SF-36), Disability of the Arm, Shoulder, and Hand (DASH), Boston Carpal Tunnel Questionnaire (BQ, also known as CTQ), the Michigan Hand Outcomes Questionnaire (MHQ), Stothard and Kamath questionnaire.

The SF-36 is a validated measure for patients' functional health and quality of life, to assess the extent to which patients' day-to-day life is affected by their health.[54] It includes 8 domains: physical functioning; social functioning; role limitations caused by physical functioning; role limitations caused by emotional problems, energy and vitality; mental health; bodily pain; and general perception of health.[55] Although it is a general health assessment questionnaire and is not sensitive enough to evaluate regional conditions,[13] SF-36 is used in combination with other region-specific questionnaires to evaluate peripheral nerve injury. In Novak and colleagues' study,[10] SF-36 bodily pain is proved to be a predictor of the DASH score, indicating that long-term disability in patients after nerve injury can be predicted by more pain. Other studies used SF-36 to evaluate functional outcome by assessing quality of life.[11,54]

The DASH questionnaire is designed to measure disability for any region of the upper extremity and can be used for single or multiple disorders.[56] It consists of 30 core questions and an optional additional 8 questions assessing work, sports, and performing arts activities, with a higher score indicating more disability.[56] The DASH score is a subjective instrument to estimate the patient's view of disability.[57] It is used for evaluation of brachial plexus surgery,[11,58,59] nerve transfer, peripheral neuroma surgery,[60] nerve repair,[11] carpal tunnel release,[61] and ulnar nerve transposition.[62] The QuickDASH was developed in 2005 to minimize time and responder burden.[63] It showed reliability, validity, and responsiveness when used for patients with either a proximal or distal disorder of the upper extremity. Compared with DASH, it is a more efficient version and retains its measurement properties.[63]

The BQ (Levine and Katz questionnaire) is a self-administered questionnaire for the assessment of severity of symptoms and functional status in patients who have CTS.[64] It consists of subscales of symptom severity and functional status. The first scale includes 11 questions of pain, altered sensibility, and weakness. The second assesses the patient's self-reported ability to perform 8 tasks.[56] It has been shown to be useful in quantifying severity of symptoms and functional state of patients before and after surgery. However, it was not possible to predict the outcome results in CTS from the preoperative scores, because there was no statistically significant relationship between them.[65] A study indicates that BQ score at 2 weeks is a reliable, responsive, and practical instrument for outcome measure in carpal tunnel surgery, and it is equivalent to 6 months postoperative score.[66] The questionnaire has also been used to identify potential prognostic factors influencing outcome[47] and to predict scar pain after carpal tunnel release.[67] In relation to objective measurements, both scales had a positive, but modest or weak, correlation with 2PD and Semmes-Weinstein monofilament testing,[64] and no relation with nerve conduction studies preoperatively and postoperatively.[65,68,69] Some investigators recommend that BQ and nerve conduction data should be used together to monitor patients with CTS.[65]

The MHQ is a 37-item self-assessment instrument, which measures disability along 6 domains: function, activities of daily living, pain, hand appearance, patient satisfaction, and work disability.[70] It is used to assess different hand disorders, including CTS. In assessing CTS, the MHQ is more specific than the DASH, because it has questions relating only to the hand, and can measure symptom and function separately. It is more versatile than BQ but also less specific, because questions relating to pain are not phrased explicitly for CTS, such as tingling and numbness. The MHQ may be more useful when independent scores from multiple domains are required or when comparison with an unaffected control hand is needed. A study also revealed that the MHQ might be more sensitive to functional changes; the DASH seems more correlated with disability days.[71]

SUMMARY

Because of the complexities of neurophysiology, assessment of recovery after peripheral nerve surgery remains a complex process for therapists and surgeons. A combination of tests, which correlate with neurophysiologic parameters and integrated hand function, is required to provide a valid, reproducible, and comprehensive assessment of outcomes. Measurement instruments for peripheral nerve surgery generally include sensory tests, motor function tests, integrated hand function tests, pain and discomfort assessments, neurophysiologic outcome measurements, and patient-reported outcomes. With a plethora of tests to choose from, researchers need to focus on measurements best relevant to specific conditions and research questions. These data will help researchers have a better understanding of the recovery process and provide the best possible outcomes for the patients.

REFERENCES

1. Epstein AM. The outcomes movement–will it get us where we want to go? N Engl J Med 1990;323: 266–70.
2. Chung KC, Burns PB, Davis Sears E. Outcomes research in hand surgery: where have we been and where should we go? J Hand Surg Am 2006; 31:1373–9.
3. Relman AS. Assessment and accountability: the third revolution in medical care. N Engl J Med 1988;319:1220–2.
4. Waljee JF, Chung KC. Outcomes research in rheumatoid arthritis. Hand Clin 2011;27:115–26.
5. Greenfield S. The state of outcome research: are we on target? N Engl J Med 1989;320:1142–3.
6. Lundborg G. A 25-year perspective of peripheral nerve surgery: evolving neuroscientific concepts and clinical significance. J Hand Surg Am 2000; 25:391–414.
7. Scholz T, Krichevsky A, Sumarto A, et al. Peripheral nerve injuries: an international survey of current treatments and future perspectives. J Reconstr Microsurg 2009;25:339–44.
8. Taylor CA, Braza D, Rice JB, et al. The incidence of peripheral nerve injury in extremity trauma. Am J Phys Med Rehabil 2008;87:381–5.
9. Rosen B. Recovery of sensory and motor function after nerve repair. A rationale for evaluation. J Hand Ther 1996;9:315–27.
10. Novak CB, Anastakis DJ, Beaton DE, et al. Patient-reported outcome after peripheral nerve injury. J Hand Surg Am 2009;34:281–7.
11. Ahmed-Labib M, Golan JD, Jacques L. Functional outcome of brachial plexus reconstruction after trauma. Neurosurgery 2007;61:1016–22 [discussion: 22–3].
12. Choi PD, Novak CB, Mackinnon SE, et al. Quality of life and functional outcome following brachial plexus injury. J Hand Surg Am 1997;22:605–12.
13. Kitajima I, Doi K, Hattori Y, et al. Evaluation of quality of life in brachial plexus injury patients after reconstructive surgery. Hand Surg 2006;11: 103–7.
14. Jerosch-Herold C. Measuring outcome in median nerve injuries. J Hand Surg Br 1993;18:624–8.
15. Bell-Krotoski J, Tomancik E. The repeatability of testing with Semmes-Weinstein monofilaments. J Hand Surg Am 1987;12:155–61.
16. Imai H, Tajima T, Natsuma Y. Interpretation of cutaneous pressure threshold (Semmes-Weinstein monofilament measurement) following median nerve repair and sensory reeducation in the adult. Microsurgery 1989;10:142–4.
17. Shooter D. Use of two-point discrimination as a nerve repair assessment tool: preliminary report. ANZ J Surg 2005;75:866–8.

18. Shimokata H, Kuzuya F. Two-point discrimination test of the skin as an index of sensory aging. Gerontology 1995;41:267–72.

19. Dellon AL. The moving two-point discrimination test: clinical evaluation of the quickly adapting fiber/receptor system. J Hand Surg Am 1978;3: 474–81.

20. Menier C, Forget R, Lambert J. Evaluation of two-point discrimination in children: reliability, effects of passive displacement and voluntary movements. Dev Med Child Neurol 1996;38:523–37.

21. Lundborg G, Rosen B. The two-point discrimination test–time for a re-appraisal? J Hand Surg Br 2004; 29:418–22.

22. Dellon ES, Mourey R, Dellon AL. Human pressure perception values for constant and moving one- and two-point discrimination. Plast Reconstr Surg 1992;90:112–7.

23. Rosen B, Lundborg G. A model instrument for the documentation of outcome after nerve repair. J Hand Surg Am 2000;25:535–43.

24. Marsh D. The validation of measures of outcome following suture of divided peripheral nerves supplying the hand. J Hand Surg Br 1990;15:25–34.

25. Haug A, Bartels A, Kotas J, et al. Sensory recovery 1 year after bridging digital nerve defects with collagen tubes. J Hand Surg Am 2013;38:90–7.

26. Ozkan T, Ozer K, Gulgonen A. Restoration of sensibility in irreparable ulnar and median nerve lesions with use of sensory nerve transfer: long-term follow-up of 20 cases. J Hand Surg Am 2001;26:44–51.

27. Medical Research Council. Nerve injuries committee: results of nerve suture. In: Seddon HJ, editor. Peripheral nerve injuries. London: Her Majesty's Stationery Office; 1954.

28. Novak CB, Kelly L, Mackinnon SE. Sensory recovery after median nerve grafting. J Hand Surg Am 1992;17:59–68.

29. Moberg E. Objective methods for determining the functional value of sensibility in the hand. J Bone Joint Surg Br 1958;40:454–76.

30. Sollerman C, Ejeskar A. Sollerman hand function test. A standardised method and its use in tetraplegic patients. Scand J Plast Reconstr Surg Hand Surg 1995;29:167–76.

31. Brandsma JW, Schreuders TA, Birke JA, et al. Manual muscle strength testing: intraobserver and interobserver reliabilities for the intrinsic muscles of the hand. J Hand Ther 1995;8:185–90.

32. Geere J, Chester R, Kale S, et al. Power grip, pinch grip, manual muscle testing or thenar atrophy–which should be assessed as a motor outcome after carpal tunnel decompression? A systematic review. BMC Musculoskelet Disord 2007;8:114.

33. Novak CB, Anastakis DJ, Beaton DE, et al. Relationships among pain disability, pain intensity, illness intrusiveness, and upper extremity disability in patients with traumatic peripheral nerve injury. J Hand Surg Am 2010;35:1633–9.

34. Badalamente M, Coffelt L, Elfar J, et al. Measurement scales in clinical research of the upper extremity, part 1: general principles, measures of general health, pain, and patient satisfaction. J Hand Surg Am 2013;38:401–6.

35. Melzack R. The McGill Pain Questionnaire: major properties and scoring methods. Pain 1975;1: 277–99.

36. Macdermid JC, Richards RS, Roth JH, et al. Endoscopic versus open carpal tunnel release: a randomized trial. J Hand Surg Am 2003;28:475–80.

37. Pollard CA. Preliminary validity study of the pain disability index. Percept Mot Skills 1984;59:974.

38. McCabe SJ, Mizgala C, Glickman L. The measurement of cold sensitivity of the hand. J Hand Surg Am 1991;16:1037–40.

39. Carlsson I, Cederlund R, Hoglund P, et al. Hand injuries and cold sensitivity: reliability and validity of cold sensitivity questionnaires. Disabil Rehabil 2008;30:1920–8.

40. Ruijs AC, Jaquet JB, Daanen HA, et al. Cold intolerance of the hand measured by the CISS questionnaire in a normative study population. J Hand Surg Br 2006;31:533–6.

41. Carlsson IK, Nilsson JA, Dahlin LB. Cut-off value for self-reported abnormal cold sensitivity and predictors for abnormality and severity in hand injuries. J Hand Surg Eur Vol 2010;35:409–16.

42. Harper CM. Preoperative and intraoperative electrophysiologic assessment of brachial plexus injuries. Hand Clin 2005;21:39–46, vi.

43. Jablecki CK, Andary MT, Floeter MK, et al. Practice parameter: electrodiagnostic studies in carpal tunnel syndrome. Report of the American Association of Electrodiagnostic Medicine, American Academy of Neurology, and the American Academy of Physical Medicine and Rehabilitation. Neurology 2002; 58:1589–92.

44. Higgs PE, Edwards DF, Martin DS, et al. Relation of preoperative nerve-conduction values to outcome in workers with surgically treated carpal tunnel syndrome. J Hand Surg Am 1997;22:216–21.

45. Bronson J, Beck J, Gillet J. Provocative motor nerve conduction testing in presumptive carpal tunnel syndrome unconfirmed by traditional electrodiagnostic testing. J Hand Surg Am 1997;22: 1041–6.

46. Padua L, Pazzaglia C, Caliandro P, et al. Carpal tunnel syndrome: ultrasound, neurophysiology, clinical and patient-oriented assessment. Clin Neurophysiol 2008;119:2064–9.

47. Gong HS, Oh JH, Bin SW, et al. Clinical features influencing the patient-based outcome after carpal tunnel release. J Hand Surg Am 2008;33:1512–7.

48. Bland JD. A neurophysiological grading scale for carpal tunnel syndrome. Muscle Nerve 2000;23:1280–3.

49. Itsubo T, Uchiyama S, Momose T, et al. Electrophysiological responsiveness and quality of life (QuickDASH, CTSI) evaluation of surgically treated carpal tunnel syndrome. J Orthop Sci 2009;14:17–23.

50. Yamano Y. Electrophysiological study of nerve grafting. J Hand Surg Am 1982;7:588–92.

51. Matsuzaki H, Yoshizu T, Maki Y, et al. Long-term clinical and neurologic recovery in the hand after surgery for severe cubital tunnel syndrome. J Hand Surg Am 2004;29:373–8.

52. Svernlov B, Larsson M, Rehn K, et al. Conservative treatment of the cubital tunnel syndrome. J Hand Surg Eur Vol 2009;34:201–7.

53. Zheng MX, Xu WD, Qiu YQ, et al. Phrenic nerve transfer for elbow flexion and intercostal nerve transfer for elbow extension. J Hand Surg Am 2010;35:1304–9.

54. Dolan RT, Butler JS, Murphy SM, et al. Health-related quality of life and functional outcomes following nerve transfers for traumatic upper brachial plexus injuries. J Hand Surg Eur Vol 2012;37:642–51.

55. McHorney CA, Ware JE Jr, Raczek AE. The MOS 36-Item Short-Form Health Survey (SF-36): II. Psychometric and clinical tests of validity in measuring physical and mental health constructs. Med Care 1993;31:247–63.

56. Smith MV, Calfee RP, Baumgarten KM, et al. Upper extremity-specific measures of disability and outcomes in orthopaedic surgery. J Bone Joint Surg Am 2012;94:277–85.

57. Vordemvenne T, Langer M, Ochman S, et al. Long-term results after primary microsurgical repair of ulnar and median nerve injuries. A comparison of common score systems. Clin Neurol Neurosurg 2007;109:263–71.

58. Kretschmer T, Ihle S, Antoniadis G, et al. Patient satisfaction and disability after brachial plexus surgery. Neurosurgery 2009;65:A189–96.

59. Liu Y, Lao J, Gao K, et al. Functional outcome of nerve transfers for traumatic global brachial plexus avulsion. Injury 2013;44(5):655–60.

60. Guse DM, Moran SL. Outcomes of the surgical treatment of peripheral neuromas of the hand and forearm: a 25-year comparative outcome study. Ann Plast Surg 2012. [Epub ahead of print].

61. Kadzielski J, Malhotra LR, Zurakowski D, et al. Evaluation of preoperative expectations and patient satisfaction after carpal tunnel release. J Hand Surg Am 2008;33:1783–8.

62. Fitzgerald BT, Dao KD, Shin AY. Functional outcomes in young, active duty, military personnel after submuscular ulnar nerve transposition. J Hand Surg Am 2004;29:619–24.

63. Beaton DE, Wright JG, Katz JN. Development of the QuickDASH: comparison of three item-reduction approaches. J Bone Joint Surg Am 2005;87:1038–46.

64. Levine DW, Simmons BP, Koris MJ, et al. A self-administered questionnaire for the assessment of severity of symptoms and functional status in carpal tunnel syndrome. J Bone Joint Surg Am 1993;75:1585–92.

65. Mondelli M, Reale F, Sicurelli F, et al. Relationship between the self-administered Boston questionnaire and electrophysiological findings in follow-up of surgically-treated carpal tunnel syndrome. J Hand Surg Br 2000;25:128–34.

66. Mallick A, Clarke M, Kershaw CJ. Comparing the outcome of a carpal tunnel decompression at 2 weeks and 6 months. J Hand Surg Am 2007;32:1154–8.

67. Kim JK, Kim YK. Predictors of scar pain after open carpal tunnel release. J Hand Surg Am 2011;36:1042–6.

68. Green TP, Tolonen EU, Clarke MR, et al. The relationship of pre- and postoperative median and ulnar nerve conduction measures to a self-administered questionnaire in carpal tunnel syndrome. Neurophysiol Clin 2012;42:231–9.

69. Heybeli N, Kutluhan S, Demirci S, et al. Assessment of outcome of carpal tunnel syndrome: a comparison of electrophysiological findings and a self-administered Boston questionnaire. J Hand Surg Br 2002;27:259–64.

70. Chung KC, Pillsbury MS, Walters MR, et al. Reliability and validity testing of the Michigan Hand Outcomes Questionnaire. J Hand Surg Am 1998;23:575–87.

71. Horng YS, Lin MC, Feng CT, et al. Responsiveness of the Michigan Hand Outcomes Questionnaire and the disabilities of the arm, shoulder, and hand questionnaire in patients with hand injury. J Hand Surg Am 2010;35:430–6.

72. Leechavengvongs S, Ngamlamiat K, Malungpaishrope K, et al. End-to-side radial sensory to median nerve transfer to restore sensation and relieve pain in C5 and C6 nerve root avulsion. J Hand Surg Am 2011;36:209–15.

73. Carlsen BT, Kircher MF, Spinner RJ, et al. Comparison of single versus double nerve transfers for elbow flexion after brachial plexus injury. Plast Reconstr Surg 2011;127:269–76.

74. Vranceanu AM, Jupiter JB, Mudgal CS, et al. Predictors of pain intensity and disability after minor hand surgery. J Hand Surg Am 2010;35:956–60.

75. Jensen MP, Karoly P, Braver S. The measurement of clinical pain intensity: a comparison of six methods. Pain 1986;27:117–26.

76. Terzis JK, Konofaos P. Radial nerve injuries and outcomes: our experience. Plast Reconstr Surg 2011;127:739–51.

77. Galanakos SP, Zoubos AB, Johnson EO, et al. Outcome models in peripheral nerve repair: time for a reappraisal or for a novel? Microsurgery 2012;32:326–33.

78. MacDermid JC. Measurement of health outcomes following tendon and nerve repair. J Hand Ther 2005;18:297–312.

79. Mc GA. The results of transposition of the ulnar nerve for traumatic ulnar neuritis. J Bone Joint Surg Br 1950;32:293–301.

Timing and Appropriate Use of Electrodiagnostic Studies

Erik R. Bergquist, MD, Warren C. Hammert, MD*

KEYWORDS

- Electrodiagnostic study • Nerve conduction study • Electromyography • Nerve injury
- Nerve compression • Carpal tunnel syndrome • Cubital tunnel syndrome • Indications

KEY POINTS

- Electrodiagnostic studies (EDS) consist of nerve conduction studies (NCS) and electromyography (EMG).
- Both NCS and EMG are needed to perform a complete electrodiagnostic study.
- Specific changes in EDS are used to characterize nerve pathology.
- Nerve injury and healing can be monitored with EDS, which provides variable information at differing time intervals.
- EDS is recommended by multidisciplinary groups in the diagnosis of carpal tunnel syndrome, yet this remains controversial.
- Prognostic information regarding mononeuropathy and polyneuropathy can be determined with EDS.
- EDS should not be used to diagnose radiculopathy.

Electrodiagnostic studies (EDS) are powerful tools used to objectively examine the physiologic status of a nerve. These consist of nerve conduction studies (NCS), which directly examine motor and sensory function of the nerve, and electromyography (EMG), which examines motor unit, action and spontaneous potentials in the muscle. Together these studies enable characterization, localization, and duration of nerve pathology and healing. An understanding of the appropriate timing and use of EDS is essential in the application of these diagnostic studies.

BASICS OF EDS

EDS consist of two components: NCS and needle EMG. These studies are used in concert to characterize and localize a pathologic lesion in a peripheral nerve. Each set of tests provides critical data, making both tests necessary to fully understand the condition.

Nerve Conduction Studies

NCS consists of stimulating a peripheral nerve and recording the response elsewhere on the nerve or associated muscle using a recording electrode.[1] Measurements are only as good as the examiner in making approximations of the locations of the nerve and its target. As a result, testing proximal and deeper structures is more challenging. When a nerve is stimulated, it is important that all elements of the nerve are depolarized. This is achieved by successively increasing the levels of current until the recorded potentials no longer increase despite an increasing stimulus. A continued increase in stimulus can result in stimulation of surrounding nerves and false recordings. The recording electrodes consist of an active and

---

Disclosure: None pertaining to this work.
Department of Orthopaedic Surgery, University of Rochester Medical Center, 601 Elmwood Avenue, Box 665, Rochester, NY 14642, USA
* Corresponding author.
E-mail address: Warren_Hammert@URMC.Rochester.edu

Hand Clin 29 (2013) 363–370
http://dx.doi.org/10.1016/j.hcl.2013.04.005
0749-0712/13/$ – see front matter © 2013 Elsevier Inc. All rights reserved.

inactive electrode placed a known distance from each other. The recorded potentials are measured as a function of time and voltage, and compared with laboratory normative values or published normal values.[2]

NCS can be divided into motor and sensory studies. Motor conduction studies are performed by placing the active recording electrode over the muscle belly and inactive recording electrode over the insertion of the muscle with the stimulation occurring over at least two points on the motor nerve. The recorded potential in the muscle represents the summated depolarization of all the muscle fibers innervated by the nerve called the compound muscle action potential (CMAP). The CMAP waveform is broken into many parts, including amplitude, latency, and conduction velocity. The amplitude is measured from the baseline to the negative peak, time from stimulation to initial deflection of the waveform is latency, and the difference in latency between proximal and distal sites of stimulation divided by the distance between those sites is conduction velocity.

The deep nature of the brachial plexus and cervical spine makes NCS difficult to perform on nerves and nerve structures in this region, given the importance of precise placement of the stimulating and recording electrodes. One additional study can be performed examining for a second CMAP called the F wave. This CMAP is created by the stimulation of a small number of anterior horn cells from the antidromic (the action potential that runs in the opposite direction from native transmission) action potential created at the time of nerve stimulation. This CMAP is much smaller with a greater latency allowing for it to be differentiated from the initial CMAP. The characteristics of the F wave can be analyzed and compared with normative values identifying pathologic features of proximal nerves and nerve structures.

Sensory studies can be performed as isolated studies or as part of a mixed nerve study. In a mixed study, the nerve of investigation creates motor and sensory action potentials when stimulated. The sensory nerve action potentials (SNAP) are measured in a similar fashion to the CMAP, except the two recording electrodes are placed over the nerve of interest instead of a muscle belly. There are marked technical differences between these two studies. SNAPs can be performed in the orthodromic or antidromic direction. Sensory axons have greater variability in the size and myelination compared with motor axons, which are more uniform.[3] Additionally, the volume of tissue (the nerve as compared with a muscle belly) stimulated is much smaller making the amplitude much smaller, and thus a greater signal-to-noise ratio.

This makes clear results more challenging to identify.

Needle EMG

Needle EMG records electrical signals in motor units within muscles by inserting a recording electrode into a muscle. EMG waveforms are divided into spontaneous and voluntary waveforms. Spontaneous waveforms are action potentials recorded on insertion of the needle, with needle movement, and at rest. Voluntary waveforms are created by voluntary muscle contraction. Differences in waveforms help to localize and characterize pathologic changes.[4]

Spontaneous waveforms relevant to hand surgery include insertional activity, fasiculation potentials, fibrillation potentials, myotonic discharges, complex repetitive discharges, myokymic discharges, neuromyotonic discharges, cramp potentials, and synkinesis. Each has a characteristic waveform and associations with normal function or pathology.

Voluntary motor unit potentials (MUP) are the action potentials recorded from motor units innervated by a single anterior horn cell. They occur in a semirhythmic pattern with specific identifiable characteristics to the appearance of the waveform. These include the duration, amplitude, and number of turns or phases (ie, the number of times the action potential crosses the baseline plus one). Multiple variables contribute to the appearance of the MUP other than pathology. These include the patient's age, muscles studied, needle position within the muscle, temperature, and strength of activation.

NERVE INJURY AND TRAUMA

Nerve repair occurs by three mechanisms: (1) remyelination, (2) collateral sprouting from preserved axons, and (3) regeneration from the site of injury. In a neuropraxic injury, the axon is intact but there is focal demyelination. Remyelination begins almost immediately on removal of the offending agent, with recovery ranging hours to months. If axonotmesis occurs, the severed axons seal over and the stump swells because of anterograde axonal transport within hours, and fragmentation and digestion of axons and myelin begin in the first few days. If less than 30% of the axons are injured, collateral sprouting occurs by Day 4 with axons traversing the segment and rearrange by Days 8 to 15. Complete healing takes 2 to 6 months. If more than 90% of axons are injured, the distal nerve segment disintegrates by wallerian degeneration and regeneration occurs from the proximal nerve end at the site of injury.[5] Injuries with 30%

to 90% may have a combination of collateral sprouting and regeneration with variability depending on the severity of injury.

Multiple transcription factors are involved in nerve regeneration. The regenerating nerve grows from a specialized growth cone at a rate of approximately 1 mm per day with improved healing rates in younger patients and more proximal lesions.[6] Muscles distal to the site of injury regain innervation sequentially as the recovering nerve reaches the end target. Motor function depends on the integrity of the muscle when the axon reaches the muscle, with muscles remaining viable for 18 to 24 months. The motor end plate begins to degenerate after the injury (because of lack of innervation) and after 24 months, the denervated muscle becomes fibrotic. Sensory nerve injuries, however, do not have a time limit for recovery or reinnervation.

Electrodiagnostic Changes in Neuropraxia

In neuropraxic lesions, the CMAP on NCS changes immediately after injury. An amplitude loss of 20% over a 25-cm distance or less indicates an injury at that site.[1] Conduction velocity decreases across the lesion because of loss of myelination and saltatory conduction on the faster conducting myelinated fibers. Conduction block may be present initially. Stimulation below the level of injury is always normal because there is no axonal loss or wallerian degeneration. The SNAP on NCS shows a decrease in amplitude across the segment, although this is difficult to measure given a natural decrease in amplitude because distance increases from the site of stimulation of up to 70%. Reduced recruitment is also found on EMG. Neuropraxia shows no changes in waveforms including duration, amplitude, phases, or spontaneous potentials (**Tables 1** and **2**).

Electrodiagnostic Changes in Axonotmesis and Neurotmesis

Axonotmesis and neurotmesis are electrodiagnostically similar, because differences between these lesions are in the support structures, not in electrophysiologic function. NCS shows a conduction block across the lesion caused by axonal and myelin sheath injury. Initially, a normal CMAP and SNAP can be identified distal to the lesion, because the axons remain in continuity distal to the lesion. In more proximal lesions, SNAPs can differentiate between preganglionic (nerve root) and postganglionic (brachial plexus) injuries. In incomplete lesions (axonotmesis), decreased recruitment is initially found on EMG. As axonal regrowth begins, increased amplitude and polyphasicity is found on EMG. In complete lesions (neurotmesis), wallerian degeneration begins distal to the lesion by the third day postinjury. The CMAP and SNAP are lost distal to the site of injury and changes develop in the spontaneous potentials as fibrillation potentials develop in the denervated muscles. As reinnervation occurs, unstable MUPs, polyphasic waveforms, and increased duration of the MUP are found in the reinnervated muscle on EMG. With nerve healing, the fibrillation potentials, unstable MUPs, and polyphasic waveforms resolve but the prolonged duration remains. For neurotmesis, reinnervation does not occur without surgical intervention to coapt the nerve ends or create a path for the nerve to follow by a conduit. The nerve heals in a fashion similar to axonotmesis with successful surgery (see **Tables 1** and **2**).

Timing of EDS

Appropriate timing of EDS varies by clinical circumstances. In situations where it is important to define a lesion early, EDS from 7 to 10 days

Table 1
Summary of NCS changes seen with axonal loss and demyelination

	Amplitude	Conduction Velocity	Distal Latency
Axonal loss	Decreased	Generally preserved Mild slowing may be seen with prominent axonal loss	Generally preserved Mild prolongation may be seen with prominent axonal loss
Demyelination	Preserved with uniform demyelination May be decreased with temporal dispersion or conduction block	Significant slowing	Significant prolongation

Table 2
Typical evolution of needle EMG findings after acute neurogenic disorder

Time for Injury	Spontaneous Activity or Fibrillations	Recruitment	Stability	Turns or Phases	Duration
1–10 d	Normal	Reduced	Stable	Normal	Normal
11–15 d	Increased	Reduced	Stable	Normal	Normal
16 d–1 mo	Fibrillations	Reduced	Stable	Turns	Mildly long
1–2 mo	Fibrillations	Reduced	Unstable	Polyphasic	Long
2–6 mo	Normal (fibrillations if incomplete reinnervation)	Reduced	Stable or unstable	Polyphasic	Long
>6 mo	Normal (fibrillations if incomplete reinnervation)	Reduced	Stable	Normal or ployphasic	Long

Reprinted from Rubin DI. Needle electromyography: basic concepts and patterns of abnormalities. Neurol Clin 2012;30(2):429–56; with permission from Elsevier, Copyright 2012.

(immediate) can localize the lesion and differentiate neurotmesis and conduction block from axonotmesis and neurotmesis. For example, in a sharp nerve laceration, although clinical examination may be sufficient, immediate EDS can assist in determining appropriate surgical action. EDS at 3 to 4 weeks (early) provides much greater information than earlier testing. It can confirm the level of the lesion, degree of nerve injury, and allow for examination of changes in the spontaneous waveforms. In neurotmesis, surgical intervention is indicated. This often requires nerve grafting or use of a conduit because nerve ends are contracted and scarred, and resection of the injured fascicles results in a gap.[7] Incomplete lesions (even a single MUP) should not be explored at this time, because intrinsic nerve healing may continue.[8,9] EDS at 2 to 6 months (intermediate) provides further information regarding nerve healing. If no further healing can be identified, or the patient has significant limitations, surgical intervention is indicated.[10] This information is helpful in determining the prognosis, and the need for other interventions in more proximal lesions. The prognosis for motor recovery depends on the distance of the lesion to the end target muscles given that nerve regeneration occurs at 1 mm per day and irreversible muscle fibrosis occurs between 18 and 24 months. There is no time limit on recovery of function for a sensory nerve. EDS at 6 to 9 months can be beneficial to monitor recovery of an incomplete nerve injury or surgically repaired nerve.

MEDIAN NERVE NEUROPATHY
Carpal Tunnel Syndrome

Carpal tunnel syndrome (CTS) is the most common entrapment neuropathy seen in the electrodiagnostic laboratory. An epidemiologic study from Sweden found the lifetime risk to be just under 10%.[11] Although EDS can objectively diagnosis CTS, the results of the test may not correspond with clinical symptoms and treatment should be based on a combination of patient history, physical examination, and EDS. Patients typically report paresthesias and numbness in the hand and radial three digits, but may state the entire hand feels numb. Symptoms proximal to the wrist are concerning for another diagnosis but may be present in 20% to 40% of patients with CTS.[12] The clinical examination, including Phalen test, Tinel sign, and median nerve (carpal tunnel) compression test, has variable sensitivity and specificity depending on the study (**Table 3**).[13] Combining these tests with more than one positive test or sign may improve sensitivity and specificity.[14] The Katz Hand Diagram found a sensitivity of 80% and specificity of 90%.[15] The American Academy of Orthopedic Surgeons (AAOS) endorses a protocol outlined by the American Association of Electrodiagnostic Medicine (AAEM),[16] which provides a standardization for performing EDS in CTS, not only in diagnosing CTS but also in identifying other pathologic lesions. Performing EDS in management of patients suspected to

Table 3
Sensitivity and specificity of the clinical examination for CTS

	Sensitivity	Specificity
Phalen test	0.46–0.80	0.51–0.91
Tinel sign	0.28–0.73	0.44–0.95
Median nerve compression test	0.04–0.79	0.25–0.96

have CTS based on history and physical examination should follow these guidelines.

NCS has been used to support the diagnosis of CTS found on history and physical examination, but it also has limitations. According to the guidelines set by the AAEM, and endorsed by the American Academy of Neurology and the American Academy of Physical Medicine and Rehabilitation, a marked variability in sensitivity and specificity has been identified over several tests used to diagnose CTS.[16] Those EDS studied range from a pooled sensitivity of 0.56 to 0.85 and pooled specificity of 0.94 to 0.99 with the outlier test, sympathetic skin response, with respective pooled sensitivity and specificity of 0.04 and 0.52. Despite the higher sensitivity and specificity rates of EDS compared with history and physical examination, it alone is not the gold standard for the diagnosis of CTS because of its overdiagnosis in asymptomatic patients and underdiagnosis of symptomatic patients.[17] In a cohort of asymptomatic workers incidentally found to have median neuropathy at the wrist, 75% did not develop symptoms of CTS at 11-year follow-up.[18] Additionally, given the sensitivity of 85%, 15% of patients with clinical CTS are electrodiagnostically negative. Finally, there are no set values to define an abnormal test on EDS.[19] Thus, the definition of a positive or negative test is left up to the standards set by the laboratory performing the study.

Benefits other than confirmation of the diagnosis of CTS have been proposed for EDS. These include diagnosis of a pathologic process other than CTS, diagnosis of a superimposed pathologic process, identifying the severity and prognosis of pathologic lesions, and to provide baseline values for comparison after an intervention.[20,21] Although the benefits of identifying other pathology are not disputed, controversy exists over defining severity because patient symptoms and electrodiagnostic values do not correlate and improvement in these values and patient symptoms are variable.[22,23]

Multidisciplinary groups have stated that EDS should be performed before performing an invasive procedure, such as surgery.[16,24] These studies site the correlation between clinical presentation, EDS, and good surgical outcomes. The association between clinical presentation alone or EDS alone and a good surgical outcome was not statistically significant in their analyses. Controversy ensued, citing potential harm to patients with CTS that are electrodiagnostically negative.[25] A systematic review of the benefit of EDS in the outcomes of surgery found no benefit to patients with "clear-cut clinical CTS."[26] Additionally, there is an increased cost to the health care system if all patients with suspected CTS are required to have EDS before a surgical intervention, especially if EDS provides no added value to the clinical diagnosis.[27,28]

Recurrent or Persistent Carpal Tunnel Syndrome

Although EDS is often ordered for recurrent or persistent symptoms after carpal tunnel release, the meaning is not always clear. The studies can be helpful if they are clearly worse or substantially improved because they would indicate there is worsening compression or improvement and symptoms are likely not related to persistent compression, but underlying nerve dysfunction. When the results are similar to preoperative studies, the interpretation is less clear because EDS does not return to normal after carpal tunnel release and may have minimal change with adequate decompression.[29] These are most helpful when performed by the same electromyographer who performed the original studies because this eliminates the variability between centers and individuals.[17]

Median Nerve Neuropathy in the Arm

EDS is helpful in defining median neuropathy other than CTS. Symptoms include pain in the arm, forearm, and hand with paresthesias and sensory loss in the median nerve distribution including the palmar cutaneous branch in the hand. In cases of demyelination a focal conduction block can be identified on NCS. In cases of significant axonal loss without conduction block, the lesion can not be definitively identified on NCS. EMG can be used to localize the level of the lesion. Examination of nonmedian nerve innervated muscles is critical to exclude brachial plexopathy, cervical radiculopathy, and motor neuron disease.

RADIAL NERVE NEUROPATHY

The radial nerve is the most commonly injured peripheral nerve.[30] Patient's with radial nerve injury frequently identify pain at the lesion site with weakness and a sensory deficit. Physical examination often identifies the level of injury. Those with injuries above the spiral groove present with weakness of the elbow, wrist, and finger extension, along with sensory loss over the posterior arm, forearm, and dorsolateral hand and fingers. Injuries at the spiral groove cause weakness of wrist and finger extension with sensory loss over the dorsolateral hand and fingers. Compression at the arcade of Frohse results in dysfunction to the posterior interosseous nerve, resulting in weakness of finger extension with no sensory deficit.

Injury to the superficial radial sensory branch causes no motor deficit, but instead a loss of sensation over the dorsolateral hand and fingers.

EDS has prognostic value in radial nerve trauma. Examination of nerve recovery after radial nerve injury found a recordable CMAP in the extensor indicis proprius or recruitment of brachioradialis on EMG resulted in a grade 3 or higher strength in 92% when conducted between 2 weeks and 8 months. No CMAP in the extensor indicis proprius but recruitment on EMG of brachioradialis had 65% with grade 3 or higher strength. No recruitment on EMG of brachioradialis found only 33% of patients with grade 3 or higher strength. However, 60% of patients with absent CMAP still had complete motor recovery.[31]

ULNAR NERVE NEUROPATHY

The ulnar nerve is commonly compressed at the elbow and wrist. Ulnar nerve compression at the elbow is the second most common mononeuropathy after CTS.[32] A focused examination of the hand can determine if the ulnar nerve lesion is proximal or distal to Guyon canal, involves only the superficial sensory branch, involves just the deep motor ulnar branch, or both. EDS can localize a lesion to the elbow, wrist, or area proximal to the elbow and determine if it is caused by demyelination or axonal loss.

NCS has a prognostic value in ulnar neuropathy. Conduction block at the elbow when recording the first dorsal interosseous muscle with a normal abductor digiti minimi found 86% full recovery regardless of treatment, whereas only 7% of patients had subjective recovery if there was conduction block at the first dorsal interosseous and low amplitude CMAP at the abductor digiti minimi.[33]

EDS for recurrent or persistent ulnar neuropathy is similar to recurrent or persistent CTS and has the same limitations described previously.

PERIPHERAL NEUROPATHY

Diagnosing a patient with peripheral neuropathy requires a comprehensive history and physical examination. Patient's subjective complaints of weakness and sensory loss can be challenging to diagnose, because findings on physical examination are late findings. Muscles do not become weak until the supplying nerve loses 50% of its axons and sensation is a subjective component of the examination. EDS can assist in the diagnosis and localization of peripheral neuropathy by providing objective sensory nerve data and fibrillation potentials are detected when a nerve has lost only a small number of axons. EDS determines the pathologic nerve distribution thereby helping to establish the cause of the neuropathy. It is uncommon for a peripheral neuropathy to involve predominantly the upper extremity, making it important to assess the lower extremity and rule out upper extremity mononeuropathy. The short list of upper extremity predominant peripheral neuropathy includes lead toxicity, porphyria, vasculitis, chronic inflammatory demyelinating polyneuropathy, multifocal motor neuropathy, and hereditary liability to pressure palsies.[34] These occur through injury to the axon as in vasculitis, injury to the myelin sheath as in chronic inflammatory demyelinating polyneuropathy, or the formation of dysfunctional myelin as in hereditary liability to pressure palsies.

BRACHIAL PLEXOPATHY

The superficial location of the brachial plexus makes it susceptible to trauma. Lesions are often identified in patients referred for other reasons emphasizing the need for a complete electrodiagnostic examination when studies are ordered for other reasons.[35] Brachial plexus lesions are classified as supraclavicular (roots and trunks); retroclavicular (divisions); and infraclavicular (cords and branches). Of these, supraclavicular is the most common and most severe.

Each brachial plexus element has its own muscle and SNAP domain. Injuries are categorized as demyelinating and axonal loss, similar to other nerve injuries. Brachial plexus injuries with axonal loss are most common. NCS shows decreased CMAP and SNAP amplitude with normal or decreased conduction velocity. Sensory NCS has the greatest sensitivity toward axonal loss and thus the ability to identify and localize the lesion. Motor NCS can quantify axonal loss by comparing the amplitude and negative area under the curve when compared with the contralateral side, in which the dropout of MUP is proportional to the number of axons lost. Fibrillation potentials are proportional to the number of denervated muscles. EMG may falsely localize the lesion more distal than the actual lesion. Lesions proximal to the dorsal root ganglion have motor NCS and EMG but sensory NCS only assesses postganglionic sensory fibers, which are not identifiable. The evolution, timing, and further nerve testing are similar to other nerve injuries.[35]

The prognosis after brachial plexus injury is directly related to the potential for reinnervation. If supporting structures are intact and the distance between the denervated muscles and the nerve lesion is short there is a chance for recovery.

Brachial plexus injuries with axonal loss resulting in loss of function of the intrinsic muscles of the hand are unlikely to have a good functional outcome given the time required for the axon to reach those muscles before the development of significant fibrosis within the muscle.[35]

RADICULOPATHY

EDS has limited use in radiculopathy. The most valuable findings are in patients with focal neurologic deficits found on physical examination. NCS has a low sensitivity for radiculopathy. Disk protrusion or spondylosis usually only damages a fraction of the nerve root fibers causing minimal deficits, which can be difficult to detect with NCS. Symptoms of pain and paresthesias are mediated through small C-type sensory fibers, which are too small to be studied. Additionally, the intraspinal location of most lesions makes direct NCS impossible.[36] Loss of almost 50% of motor axons is required for reliable CMAP reduction. F wave antidromic nerve stimulation has a low sensitivity for radiculopathy and is insufficient alone to make the diagnosis of radiculopathy. Correlation of EDS with radiculopathy is difficult because there is no gold standard for diagnosis of radiculopathy. When comparing EDS with magnetic resonance imaging, there was a 50%, 70%, and 67% concordance with C5, C6, and C7, respectively.[37]

CLINIC-BASED EDS FOR CTS

Simple intraoffice devices have been developed to perform NCS specifically for CTS. They provide the convenience for patients from having to see another provider to have EDS performed. Additionally, they provide a decrease in overall cost to the patient by minimizing the number of providers seen. When comparing this device with traditional EDS, it was found to be 98% specific for CTS.[38] However, these devices have limitations because they only perform sensory NCS and do not find other nerve pathologies. Therefore, they do not meet the guidelines for EDS as recommended by the AAOS or the AAEM.[13,16]

SUMMARY

EDS provides objective data regarding the status of peripheral nerves. Both NCS and EMG are required for a complete electrodiagnostic examination. EDS helps characterize the severity and location of nerve injuries, which assists in providing patient prognosis and determining treatment options. EDS can provide localization in the first few days after a nerve injury, but much greater information is provided 2 to 3 weeks after the injury after wallerian degeneration occurs. Furthermore, EDS can be used to monitor nerve healing in the months after injury. The requirement that EDS be performed before surgical intervention remains controversial for CTS. Currently, EDS is recommended by the AAOS and AAEM before surgery for CTS. EDS has been found to characterize, localize, provide prognostic information, and assist in treatment plans for brachial plexus, ulnar, and radial nerve injuries. It can assist in diagnosing peripheral neuropathy in the early stages when a clinical diagnosis proves challenging. The use of EDS in radiculopathy is limited. Finally, new clinic-based sensory NCS devices can reduce costs and have similar specificity as traditional EDS, but have limitations in that they only diagnose CTS and are not uniformly accepted.[13,16] EDS is a powerful tool, which when used with correct timing and for appropriate uses, provides important information for health care providers and improves patient care.

REFERENCES

1. Jones LK. Nerve conduction studies: basic concepts and patterns of abnormalities. Neurol Clin 2012;30(2):405–27.
2. Wang SH, Robinson LR. Considerations in reference values for nerve conduction studies. Phys Med Rehabil Clin N Am 1998;9(4):907–23, viii.
3. Wilbourn AJ. Sensory nerve conduction studies. J Clin Neurophysiol 1994;11(6):584–601.
4. Rubin DI. Needle electromyography: basic concepts and patterns of abnormalities. Neurol Clin 2012;30(2):429–56.
5. Campbell WW. Evaluation and management of peripheral nerve injury. Clin Neurophysiol 2008; 119(9):1951–65.
6. Burnett MG, Zager EL. Pathophysiology of peripheral nerve injury: a brief review. Neurosurg Focus 2004;16(5):E1.
7. Kline DG, Hackett ER. Reappraisal of timing for exploration of civilian peripheral nerve injuries. Surgery 1975;78(1):54–65.
8. Dubuisson A, Kline DG. Indications for peripheral nerve and brachial plexus surgery. Neurol Clin 1992;10(4):935–51.
9. Spinner RJ, Kline DG. Surgery for peripheral nerve and brachial plexus injuries or other nerve lesions. Muscle Nerve 2000;23(5):680–95.
10. Kline DG. Timing for exploration of nerve lesions and evaluation of the neuroma-in-continuity. Clin Orthop Relat Res 1982;163:42–9.
11. Atroshi I, Gummesson C, Johnsson R, et al. Prevalence of carpal tunnel syndrome in a general population. JAMA 1999;282(2):153–8.

12. Zanette G, Marani S, Tamburin S. Proximal pain in patients with carpal tunnel syndrome: a clinical-neurophysiological study. J Peripher Nerv Syst 2007;12(2):91–7.

13. Keith MW, Masear V, Chung K, et al. Diagnosis of carpal tunnel syndrome. J Am Acad Orthop Surg 2009;17(6):389–96.

14. Fertl E, Wöber C, Zeitlhofer J. The serial use of two provocative tests in the clinical diagnosis of carpal tunnel syndrome. Acta Neurol Scand 1998;98(5): 328–32.

15. Katz JN, Stirrat CR. A self-administered hand diagram for the diagnosis of carpal tunnel syndrome. J Hand Surg 1990;15(2):360–3.

16. Medicine E. Practice parameter for electrodiagnostic studies in carpal tunnel syndrome: summary statement. Muscle Nerve 2002;25(6):918–22.

17. Watson JC. The electrodiagnostic approach to carpal tunnel syndrome. Neurol Clin 2012;30(2): 457–78.

18. Nathan PA, Keniston RC, Myers LD, et al. Natural history of median nerve sensory conduction in industry: relationship to symptoms and carpal tunnel syndrome in 558 hands over 11 years. Muscle Nerve 1998;21(6):711–21.

19. Werner RA, Andary M. Electrodiagnostic evaluation of carpal tunnel syndrome. Muscle Nerve 2011; 44(4):597–607.

20. Boniface SJ, Morris I, Macleod A. How does neurophysiological assessment influence the management and outcome of patients with carpal tunnel syndrome? Br J Rheumatol 1994;33(12):1169–70.

21. Haupt WF, Wintzer G, Schop A, et al. Long-term results of carpal tunnel decompression. Assessment of 60 cases. J Hand Surg Br 1993;18(4):471–4.

22. Longstaff L, Milner RH, O'Sullivan S, et al. Carpal tunnel syndrome: the correlation between outcome, symptoms and nerve conduction study findings. J Hand Surg Br 2001;26(5):475–80.

23. Robinson L, Kliot M. Stop using arbitrary grading schemes in carpal tunnel syndrome. Muscle Nerve 2008;37(6):804.

24. Keith MW, Masear V, Amadio PC, et al. Treatment of carpal tunnel syndrome. J Am Acad Orthop Surg 2009;17(6):397–405.

25. Finsen V, Russwurm H. Neurophysiology not required before surgery for typical carpal tunnel syndrome. J Hand Surg Br 2001;26(1):61–4.

26. Jordan R, Carter T, Cummins C. A systematic review of the utility of electrodiagnostic testing in carpal tunnel syndrome. Br J Gen Pract 2002;52(481): 670–3.

27. Graham B. The value added by electrodiagnostic testing in the diagnosis of carpal tunnel syndrome. J Bone Joint Surg Am 2008;90(12):2587–93.

28. Zyluk A, Szlosser Z. The results of carpal tunnel release for carpal tunnel syndrome diagnosed on clinical grounds, with or without electrophysiological investigations: a randomized study. J Hand Surg Eur Vol 2013;38(1):44–9.

29. El-Hajj T, Tohme R, Sawaya R. Changes in electrophysiological parameters after surgery for the carpal tunnel syndrome. J Clin Neurophysiol 2010;27(3): 224–6.

30. Robinson LR. Traumatic injury to peripheral nerves. Suppl Clin Neurophysiol 2004;57:173–86.

31. Malikowski T, Micklesen PJ, Robinson LR. Prognostic values of electrodiagnostic studies in traumatic radial neuropathy. Muscle Nerve 2007;36(3): 364–7.

32. Dimberg EL. Electrodiagnostic evaluation of ulnar neuropathy and other upper extremity mononeuropathies. Neurol Clin 2012;30(2):479–503.

33. Friedrich JM, Robinson LR. Prognostic indicators from electrodiagnostic studies for ulnar neuropathy at the elbow. Muscle Nerve 2011;43(4):596–600.

34. Ross MA. Electrodiagnosis of peripheral neuropathy. Neurol Clin 2012;30(2):529–49.

35. Ferrante MA. Electrodiagnostic assessment of the brachial plexus. Neurol Clin 2012;30(2):551–80.

36. Levin KH. Approach to the patient with suspected radiculopathy. Neurol Clin 2012;30(2):581–604.

37. Nicotra A, Khalil NM, O'Neill K. Cervical radiculopathy: discrepancy or concordance between electromyography and magnetic resonance imaging? Br J Neurosurg 2011;25(6):789–90.

38. Tolonen U, Kallio M, Ryhänen J, et al. A handheld nerve conduction measuring device in carpal tunnel syndrome. Acta Neurol Scand 2007;115(6): 390–7.

Major Peripheral Nerve Injuries

Jonathan Isaacs, MD

KEYWORDS

- Nerve injury • Neurorrhaphy • Nerve allograft • Major peripheral nerves

KEY POINTS

- Proper use of electrodiagnostic and advanced imaging studies such as magnetic resonance imaging and ultrasound improves timely identification of appropriate surgical candidates for nerve exploration.
- Nerve injuries with an unknown zone of injury should be allowed to demarcate, and aggressive debridement of all damaged nerve tissue should be performed before repair.
- End-to-end fascicular alignment is critical to successful nerve regeneration and may be facilitated by use of nerve connectors during coaptation.
- Nerve conduits have a limited role in overcoming major peripheral nerve gaps.
- Decellularized nerve allograft is a promising reconstructive tool for major peripheral nerve repairs.

INTRODUCTION

Despite decades of advancements in peripheral nerve research, the treatment of major peripheral nerve injuries remains challenging. These injuries can be devastating to patients who often must suffer months and even years of uncertainty as they wait for the recovery that may never come. Families must remain supportive even when they do not appreciate the unique pain associated with many nerve injuries or the difficult-to-comprehend handicap that comes with loss of tactile sensation. Even the care providers (the surgeons, the therapists, and the pain management physicians) must all maintain conviction and optimism even when the perfect repair fails to progress, the recovery that should have occurred does not, and the functional return does not allow a return of function. Although positive results cannot be guaranteed, a better appreciation of the obstacles to nerve regeneration can translate to more effective treatment paradigms and repair techniques and strategies. In this way, the potential for an acceptable or even good outcome when dealing with major peripheral nerve injuries in isolation or as part of a more complex injury pattern can be maximized.

This article discusses current concepts regarding the diagnosis, treatment, and expected outcomes of injury to the median, ulnar, and radial nerves. Although the principle of expectant observation of closed nerve injuries has not changed, there has been a shift toward earlier exploration. Advances in nerve imaging technology, specifically magnetic resonance imaging (MRI)[1] and ultrasound, have also facilitated identification of ruptured nerves, which allows earlier treatment. Proper nerve repair technique continues to emphasize atraumatic handling of the nerve, tensionless approximation, and accurate alignment of fascicles. New coaptation tools such as nerve connectors can now help achieve these goals. Likewise, a growing awareness of the limitations of nerve conduits as well as the recent introduction of acellular nerve allograft has redefined the management of short nerve gaps.

Disclosure: The author has received consultant fees and has received speaking fees from AxoGen, Inc and partial research support from Integra LifeSciences, Inc.

Division of Hand Surgery, Department of Orthopaedic Surgery, Virginia Commonwealth University Health System, 1200 East Broad Street, PO Box 980153, Richmond, VA 23298, USA

E-mail address: jisaacs@mcvh-vcu.edu

hand.theclinics.com

DIAGNOSES

The identification of a significant major nerve injury is not difficult, and neurologic deficits such as complete or partial muscle paralysis and paresthesias should be diagnosed on most posttrauma examinations. The occasional miss can usually be attributed to examiner inexperience, a failure to recognize the potential for such an injury (so the proper examination is never even performed), or a sense of denial by either the examiner or the patient (the numbness is probably caused by swelling and the lack of movement caused by pain). The challenge is to identify which nerve injuries will recover on their own, and which require surgical treatment.

The answer to this question starts with an understanding of the spectrum of anatomic and physiologic effects of nerve trauma and how nerves regenerate.

UNDERSTANDING THE DECISION TREE

An injured nerve begins the regeneration process immediately following the injury. If the only damage is to the myelin sheath, complete recovery can occur, but may take 3 months. When the neural elements are disrupted, each axon forms multiple filopodia, which advance and form multiple branches toward the distal nerve stump. For an axonotmetic injury, in which the endoneural tubes are still intact, the regenerating axons progress uninhibited with an excellent chance of eventually achieving reinnervation. The length of recovery is based on an approximate regeneration rate of 1 mm/d, although this is typically faster for proximal injuries, slows as regeneration time becomes longer, and may be slower in areas of partially damaged nerve tissue in which the axons must work around scar tissue. For partial and complete internal ruptures, the axons still try to advance but become tangled in disrupted internal architecture and scar tissue and are often unable to bridge the zone of injury. Even though the nerve is technically still intact, spontaneous regeneration does not occur. A neuroma in continuity may form, in which the nerve feels firm and scarred or, conversely, the nerve may become thin and stretched out (like taffy), or even appear normal. Neuropraxic injuries recover spontaneously and neurotmesis requires surgical intervention. Axonotmetic injuries may recover spontaneously, but depend on the axons being able to regenerate uninhibited to the distal nerve stump. If it occurs, spontaneous recovery is typically better than nerve reconstruction. Adding complexity to this dilemma, more than one degree of injury (part of

the nerve can be neuropraxic and another part axonotmetic) can coexist.

MAKING THE DECISION

A patient presenting with a laceration and a neurologic deficit is presumed to have a nerve transection and surgery is recommended. There are biological and clinical implications for doing the surgery as soon as possible.[2] The insult to the nerve cell following transection of the axon is substantial and often results in cell death, which decreases the number of regenerating axons and diminishes reinnervation potential.[3] Early repair has been shown to improve axon survival,[4] although the clinical significance of this is unknown. Early surgical exploration minimizes nerve stump retraction and fibrosis,[5] as well as loss of surface landmarks. Clean lacerations repaired within a few days are typically amendable to primary repair.

Nerve injuries associated with blunt trauma, such as avulsion, tearing, or penetrating missile trauma, have a greater zone of injury and primary repair is unpredictable. Immediate surgical exploration is based on non-nerve indications, and the nerve is only exposed if accessible in the established surgical wound. For example, irrigation and debridement with open reduction and internal fixation of an open humerus fracture offers easy access to the radial nerve, which should be inspected. In contrast, median nerve exploration concurrent with treatment of an open dorsal wrist wound following a gunshot injury is not necessarily indicated. The nerve stumps of ruptured or torn nerves, if visualized, should be sutured together with a blue 2-0 prolene (or analogous stitch) to prevent excessive retraction and to facilitate delayed reconstruction. Primary repair at the time of exploration is doomed if the damaged nerve is not resected[6] and a delay to allow demarcation is recommended (**Fig. 1**). At around 3 weeks, the scarred nerve tissue can be resected and the nerve repaired secondarily. Ring and colleagues[7] reported 100% failure when ruptured radial nerves were fixed at the same time as initial treatment of associated open humerus fractures. If the nerve is intact or not visualized, further assessment should be analogous to a closed nerve injury.

For closed nerve injuries (or nerves found to be intact at early exploration) the dilemma is determining whether the nerve will regenerate on its own (neuropraxic or axonotmetic injuries) or whether the zone of injury needs to be excised and reconstructed.

The use of electrodiagnostic studies following nerve injuries is discussed elsewhere in this issue.

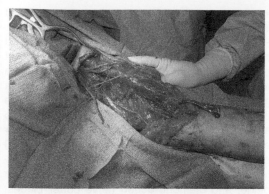

Fig. 1. Upper arm injured from animal attack. Large zone of injury would compromise nerve regeneration if repair is performed during this initial exploration.

If nerve conduction and electromyography studies are delayed until at least 3 weeks after injury, neuropraxic injuries can be differentiated, the patient reassured, and continued expectant observation recommended. Nerves that are completely ruptured or that show profound physical changes related to significant internal rupture and derangement can also be identified at this early time point using either ultrasound[8,9] or high-resolution MRI.[1] Both technologies depend on operator and interpreter proficiency. However, by identifying injuries that definitely require surgery, surgical treatment can be planned. A delay of approximately 3 weeks to allow zone of injury demarcation (similar to open ruptured nerves) is still recommended before exploration and repair.[10]

When the nerve is intact (as shown by direct inspection during non-nerve–related early surgery or visualization using ultrasound or MRI technology), many will recover spontaneously. Shao and colleagues[11] reported an almost 90% chance of spontaneous recovery in closed radial nerve injuries. Axonal regeneration progresses at approximately 1 mm/d,[12] and recovery times can be estimated by measuring from the site of the expected injury to the closest denervated muscle. The number of millimeters measured (an analogous ratio is an inch/month) should equate to the approximate number of days until clinical muscle recovery might be expected. A progressing Tinel can be helpful in following the progressive axonal march toward distal targets.

There are several caveats to this strategy:

1. The site of injury cannot always be precisely determined, especially in high-energy or multi-level trauma
2. Tinel sign, although helpful when present and well defined, is not completely reliable and can be misleading

3. Prolonged observation can be detrimental to the final outcome if axon regeneration does not occur and formal nerve reconstruction is overly delayed

DENERVATION ATROPHY OF MUSCLE AND NERVE

The loss of muscle fiber size, nucleic material, and contractile proteins temporally related to muscle denervation was recognized more than 50 years ago and has been termed denervation atrophy.[13] If reinnervation cannot be achieved by 18 months, the potential for recovery is so low that continued pursuit of this goal is not considered worthwhile. With persistent denervation, the muscle tissue is eventually replaced with fibrotic adipose tissue, which does not mean that at 18 months a biological switch is activated and reinnervation is no longer possible, but rather that, as time passes, the potential for reinnervation diminishes (by approximately 1% per week[14]) to unsalvageable levels. More recently, the progressive degeneration of neurotrophic potential in denervated nerve tissue has also been recognized. Schwann cells become less supportive, there is a loss of axon guidance signals, and distal endoneural tubes become blocked with proteoglycans.[15] Although this process seems to take longer than the changes affecting muscle, the implications for both motor and sensory nerve recovery are that:

1. Early nerve repair is preferred
2. Although greater than motor nerves, sensory nerves cannot be repaired indefinitely
3. Proximal motor or mixed nerve injuries may take so long to regenerate (>18 months), that alternate reconstructive strategies should be considered for motor reconstruction

HOW TO BALANCE URGENCY OR REPAIR AND THE DIAGNOSTIC BENEFITS OF DELAY

There needs, therefore, to be a balance between observation (to allow potential axonal regeneration) and surgical exploration (to ensure appropriate and timely repair if axonal regeneration has not progressed). A delay of 3 to 4 months in exploration allows recovery of neuropraxic injuries and would equals 75 or 100 mm (3 or 4 inches) of axonal regeneration through the zone of injury if the microneural environment is favorable for nerve regeneration. If the microenvironment is unfavorable, the unproductive regenerative efforts of the axons result in a neuroma in continuity. This physiologic rationale underlies the common clinical pattern of a baseline electromyogram (EMG) at

3 to 4 weeks after injury, with a follow-up EMG at 3 to 4 months.

If axonal regeneration is still lacking at 3 to 4 months, surgical exploration is indicated. Although occult axonal regeneration may still be occurring, the necessity of a definitive decision at this point demands a direct visual and tactile inspection of the nerve. External and internal neurolysis is performed as necessary and, when in doubt, intraoperative nerve conduction studies are performed. Sterile electrodes are placed above the zone of injury and 75 or 100 mm (3 or 4 inches) distal to the zone of injury (usually 100 mm of separation between the two electrodes is necessary to differentiate between shock artifact and a nerve action potential). The detection of a nonaveraged nerve action potential indicates the presence of axons across the zone of injury, and, as established by Tiel and colleagues,[16] suggests a 90% chance of continued nerve recovery.

Although not a guarantee, these odds are better than resecting and grafting. Patchy recovery in which some muscles are reinnervated and others (even more proximal) are not may be related to unrecognized injury to proximal nerve branches, mixed degrees of injury across the width of the nerve (one part of the nerve maintains endoneural tube continuity and another part of the nerve has more significant internal derangement), or misdirection of regenerating axons. Once this phenomenon is recognized, efforts can be directed at using nerve transfers to innervate the skipped muscles or delayed reconstructive efforts (such as muscle or tendon transfer) considered. For injuries in which the nerve is intact but intraoperative studies fail to support the presence of axonal regeneration, the zone of injury needs to be resected and reconstructed.

NERVE REPAIR

A technically perfect nerve repair must consist of 4 parts: (1) complete debridement to healthy nerve tissue, (2) nerve approximation without tension, (3) end-on alignment of fascicles, (4) atraumatic and secure mechanical coaptation of nerve ends.

DEBRIDEMENT

For sharp, clean lacerations, minimal debridement of the nerve ends is typically necessary. However, even sharp lacerations often involve an underappreciated tearing effect so more nerve tissue damage may be present than expected. Healthy nerve stumps show fascicular patterns, and the fascicles on the proximal stump should protrude. For subacute or chronic injuries, stretching or avulsing injuries, or any other injuries with a large zone of injury, substantial resection may be necessary. However, until all of the injured or compromised nerve tissue has been excised, the repair will not be successful and the temptation to compromise resection of the damaged nerve tissue to avoid a gap must be resisted. Axons do not regenerate through an area of scarred nerve sutured to another area of scarred nerve.[17] Techniques for excising the damaged nerve tissue include a #10 blade and a tongue depressor, specialty nerve-holding clamps combined with a disposable razor blade, and diamond-edged nerve cutter blades. The important aspect is to avoid crushing the nerve; scissors are typically an option only for the smallest nerves.

Nerves have an excellent blood supply, but this means that the debrided nerve stump often bleeds. The accumulation of blood between approximated nerve ends (or within a nerve conduit) theoretically increases the chance of axon impeding scar tissue formation. Hemostasis of the cut end of a nerve stump can be tricky. If the blood vessel is visualized, a microbipolar set on a low setting and applied under irrigation (to diminish the spread of thermal energy) can be done carefully with the risk of damaging the nerve tissue. As an alternative, applying epinephrine (with a pledget) to the nerve stump for several minutes can be effective. Thrombin spray or gel foam may work as well, but has the disadvantage of adding a foreign material and clot to the repair site.

NERVE APPROXIMATION

Following debridement, the size of the gap must be determined. Although small gaps can be repaired primarily by mobilizing or transposing the ends of the nerve, the temptation of pulling the ends together to avoid the time, energy, and morbidity of grafting (as well as the theoretic concerns of a second nerve suture line) must be tempered against the detrimental effects of tension on the nerve repair.[18] Tension has been shown to inhibit Schwann cell activation and axonal regeneration.[19] As little as 8% stretch on nerve tissue results in temporary ischemia, and elongation of 15% cause irreversible ischemic changes.[20,21] Ten percent stretch is generally considered acceptable[17] (although the limit may be less for a fibrotic nerve).

Judging tension at the repair site can be difficult, but a useful rule is that a single 8-0 nylon suture should be enough to maintain the coaptation. Relief of tension by joint positioning is, in general, a bad idea and predisposes to joint contractures, pain from pulling at the repair, or failure of the repair.

ALIGNMENT

Once the nerve ends can be approximated, the fascicles must be aligned. Motor axons have a greater tendency to travel down better or more neurosupportive endoneural tubes, although the mechanism by which this occurs and the net clinical effects are unknown.[22,23] Although eccentric alignment techniques such as intraoperative nerve staining[24] or awake stimulation[25] have been described, visual alignment using surface vessels and fascicular patterns is easier and equally effective.

DIRECT REPAIR

Suturing the nerve stumps together using microsurgical technique is the most common method of coaptation. Because sutures generate scar tissue, the fewest sutures capable of both coaptation and alignment should be used.[10]

EPINEURAL REPAIR

The simplest suturing technique is to place the sutures through the outer epineurium only. The shallow placement of the stitches minimizes scar tissue and is the least technically demanding. However, fascicular alignment is obtained indirectly[26] and is prone to error. The tendency is to perform this repair too tightly, resulting in a perfect-appearing outer nerve surface with bunched up, misdirected fascicles inside. The nerve ends should ideally just barely touch.

FASCICULAR REPAIR

At the opposite end of the spectrum, fascicular repair requires excision of outer and inner epineurium to expose the individual fascicles. The suture is passed through the perineurium and each fascicle is individually repaired. This technique is more time consuming and technically demanding

and has not shown superiority compared with easier techniques.[27,28]

GROUP FASCICULAR REPAIR

A hybrid between epineural and fascicular repairs, group fascicular repair takes advantage of the thickened areas of inner epineurium separating groups of fascicles (**Fig. 2**). Although less aggressive than fascicular repair, the technique still controls alignment and end-to-end approximation is better than epineural repair. In the median and ulnar nerves of the forearm where topography is consistent and well known, this repair has been shown to improve outcomes.[29]

ALTERNATIVE TECHNIQUES
Fibrin Glue

Although suturing seems to be the most widely accepted nerve repair technique, it is time consuming, technically demanding, and generates intraneural scar tissue. Fibrin glue is not approved by the US Food and Drug Administration for this application, but it is one of the more commonly used alternative techniques. Fibrin glue comes as 2 separate syringes containing the components of the clotting cascade. The contents of the syringes are simultaneously applied around the approximated nerve ends and congeal together into a firm, rubbery clot. A piece of backing (such as rubber esmarch) placed behind the nerve repair can be wrapped around the mixture as the clot forms and shapes the fibrin glue into an adhesive cylinder or cocoon around the coapted ends (**Fig. 3**). Consistency is firm enough at 3 minutes to remove the backing and to trim away excess fibrin glue material.

This technique is fast and easy. Material interposed between nerve ends does not seem to interfere with axon regeneration.[30] Alignment of the nerve stumps can be difficult to maintain while applying the fibrin glue if positioning is only

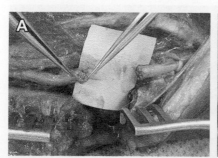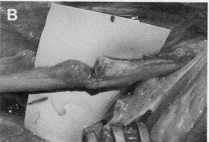

Fig. 2. Grouped fascicular repair of ulnar nerve. (*A*) Note the fascicular grouping. (*B*) Repair of motor group of fascicles; repair of remainder of nerve to follow.

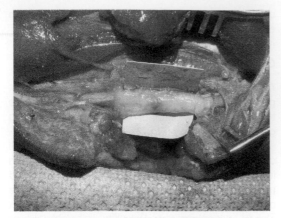

Fig. 3. Fibrin glue repair of severed nerve.

maintained with forceps, and there are concerns about the holding strength with this technique. Animal studies have noted dehisced repairs at re-exploration[31] and, when tested biomechanically, fibrin glue decreased gapping at the repair but did not add significant holding strength compared with 2 sutures alone.[32] At present, fibrin glue is primarily used as an augmenting agent to supplement suture repair.

Nerve Connectors

A more recently introduced concept, nerve connectors are short (1 cm) nerve conduits that can be used for direct primary repair. Applied in a similar manner to a conduit, each stump is pulled 4 or 5 mm into the connector. Sutures can be placed through the end of the connector and through the outer epineurium. Although sutures are still used, they are placed away from the end of the nerve stump (where axonal regeneration is occurring) and fewer of them are necessary. In addition, the tube around the repair site creates a protected microenvironment; axons are blocked from escaping, scar tissue is blocked from invading, and a concentrated neurogenic milieu

of growth factors can accumulate.[33,34] The limited amount of end-organ specificity that occurs with axonal regeneration may work better with this technique. Evans and colleagues[35] showed in a rat sciatic nerve model that a misaligned nerve repair did slightly better if repaired with a short tube than with direct suturing. Repairs using a nerve connector leave a tiny gap between the approximated nerve stumps; the fascicles are always facing each other. Although any nerve conduit can be used in this capacity, the commercially available nerve connector (AxoGen, Inc) made of porcine submucosa is ideally suited. The material is tough and flexible, transparent (approximation and alignment can be visualized), and is incorporated into the mesoneurium over time (**Figs. 4** and **5**).[36]

Gaps

Defects that cannot be overcome with mobilization need to be bridged using a conduit, allograft, or autograft.

Nerve Conduits

Although the use of conduits as nerve connectors is growing, conduits are more commonly used for overcoming short nerve gaps. The advantages described earlier for nerve connectors (protected microenvironment, and so forth[33]) are the same. The difference is that a natural fibrin clot (generated from blood serum) must form within the conduit to act as a biological bridge or scaffold between the nerve stumps.[37] Schwann cells and, subsequently, axons can then use this scaffold to migrate across the gap.[21] However, the disadvantage of this technique is that it completely depends on formation of the fibrin clot and, when this clot does not form, no nerve regeneration occurs. It is intuitive that, the longer the gap and the wider the diameter of the nerve, the less

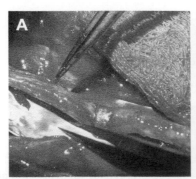
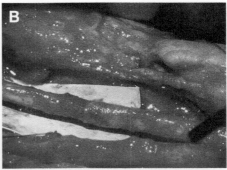

Fig. 4. Nerve connector repair of ulnar nerve. (*A*) Being sutured into place. (*B*) Completed repair.

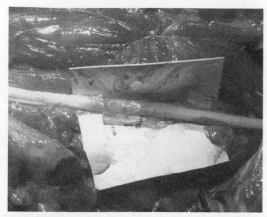

Fig. 5. Nerve connector being slid over completed repair and sutured in place to augment and support the repair.

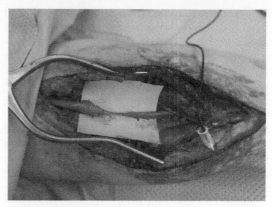

Fig. 6. Failed median nerve repair with nerve conduit. Note the inadequate nerve regeneration between stumps.

predictable the clot formation becomes, suggesting that this may not be the optimal tool for large nerves.

A recent meta-analysis offered the contrasting conclusion that conduits are as effective as autograft in bridging median and ulna nerve defects of up to 5 cm.[38] However, the data regarding nerve conduits presented in this meta-analysis are largely from case reports (level IV evidence). The 2 larger series included in the meta-analysis cover 69 patients undergoing silicone or polytetrafluoroethylene (ePTFE) conduit reconstruction of up to 6-cm gaps in median and ulnar nerves. Acceptable results were obtained with silicone bridging of gaps less than 3 cm,[39] and ePTFE conduit bridging of gaps up to 4 cm.[40] Results deteriorated with gaps longer than 3 or 4 cm. It is concerning that silicone and ePTFE conduit usage has not become more widespread following these encouraging reports more than 20 years ago and may suggest that these results were not reproducible. More recently, Chiriac and colleagues[41] published their results using polycaprolactone conduits for a variety of nerve repairs. Only 1 out of 12 major peripheral nerve repairs performed with this device resulted in an acceptable outcome. Moore and colleagues[42] published their poor results in major peripheral nerve repairs using conduits and recommended against their use in this application (**Fig. 6**).

Allograft

Acellular nerve allograft (Avance Nerve Graft; Axo-Gen, Inc, Alachua, FL) may be a better option for bridging short defects in major peripheral nerve repair. Advances in tissue processing have allowed the development of a nonimmunogenic off-the-shelf human allograft option. The preparatory process removes cells, neural debris, and chondroitin sulfate proteoglycans[43] from the graft material but leaves the remaining connective tissue architecture to act as a scaffold for nerve regeneration. Schwann cells must still migrate into the allograft from either end to support regenerating axons,[44] which may end up being a length-limiting obstacle, although in the currently available lengths this does not seem to be a problem. Chondroitin sulfate proteoglycans have been shown to inhibit axonal growth and their extraction should benefit human nerve regeneration.[45]

At present, there are no clinical studies of high-level evidence (I or II) comparing conduits, allograft, and autograft for major peripheral nerve reconstruction, so knowledge is based on comparative animal studies and level III clinical studies. Whitlock and colleagues[46] showed similar functional recovery at 3 months between isograft and acellular rat allograft repair groups in a 14-mm nerve defect. For a 28-mm graft, the isograft group showed superior functional recovery, although allograft (but not the conduit) still supported muscle reinnervation. Midgraft axonal densities and distributions were equivalent for 14-mm and 28-mm isografts and allografts, whereas conduits were markedly inferior at both lengths.[47] A similar study of only 1-cm gaps again showed equivalent histology for rat sciatic nerves repaired with allografts and isografts at 3 and 4 months after repair. Functional recovery was equivalent between these groups at 3 months, although a slight superiority was shown in the isograft group at 4 months. The conduit was inferior in all parameters at both 3-month and 4-month time points.[48]

Clinical data on major nerve repairs using allograft are limited. A multicenter registry study reported on 13 radial, ulnar, and median nerve repairs (it lacked data on 5 additional repairs).

With gap sizes ranging from 5 to 50 mm, 86% of patients achieved meaningful recovery (defined as M3–M5 or S3–S4).[49] The commercially available acellular allograft comes in diameters of up to 5 mm based on concerns of central necrosis with larger diameter sizes. Tang and colleagues[50] showed in a rodent model that matched-diameter decellularized allograft outperformed cable grafts. This finding has not been evaluated clinically but cable grafting with allograft diameters matching the cross-surface area of corresponding fascicular groups would be a reasonable approach (**Fig. 7**).

Autograft

Autograft offers neurosupportive architecture, guidance cues, neurotrophic factors, and Schwann cells, and is still the gold standard for bridging gaps in major peripheral nerve repairs. Cumulative experience with autologous nerve grafting outweighs all other techniques combined and, especially over the last 3 decades, has helped refine this technique. Graft material is derived from less important nerves harvested at the expense of some functional loss, a second surgical site, and possible donor site complications or morbidity. By harvesting a sensory nerve with a nonessential territory such as the dorsal aspect of the first web space (superficial radial nerve) or the medial side of the forearm (medial antebrachial cutaneous nerve), this trade-off is easy to rationalize. There are recent data suggesting that motor nerve graft material may be superior to sensory nerve at supporting motor axon regeneration,[51,52] but there is a limited supply of motor nerves that can be sacrificed and the potential benefit of this choice has not yet been shown. Common graft choices include the medial antebrachial cutaneous nerve, medial brachial cutaneous nerve, lateral antebrachial cutaneous nerve, superficial radial nerve, and sural nerves.

For upper extremity major nerve reconstruction, using local cutaneous nerves from the same field, especially when already nonfunctional, may seem like a particularly attractive option. However, further sacrificing sensation in a mostly insensate limb may have functional consequences. In addition, donor nerves that have been denervated for several months may be less effective in supporting axonal regeneration than freshly denervated nerve tissue.[53] For these reasons, as well as the relative ease of harvesting 30 cm or more of graft material per leg, the sural nerve is the most common source of autologous graft material for major nerve reconstruction. Sensory loss in this distribution is general well tolerated, although serious problems with neuroma formation or severe pain can occur.[54]

For major peripheral nerve reconstruction, strands of sural or other nerve graft must be stacked on each other to form a multistrand cable to cover the cross-surface area of the recipient nerve stumps. At least a 10% to 15% greater length than the measured gap should be harvested because the graft material tends to contract and preparation of the graft may waste some of the nerve tissue. Cable grafting can be performed by suturing each strand individually (and trying to match up corresponding fascicular patterns) or the cable can be constructed on the back table. The appropriate number of strands (usually 2 to 4 for median and ulnar nerves) can be stacked together and fibrin glue applied around the ends of the cable graft to hold them together. The ends of the cable graft are freshened and the excess fibrin glue can be removed. The cable can now be sutured into place, taking care to pass the suture into epineurium and not just the fibrin glue (**Fig. 8**). As an alternative, nerve

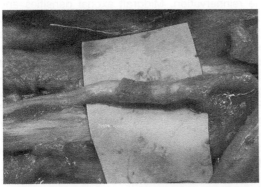

Fig. 7. Nerve cable allograft sutured into place and reinforced with a nerve connector for median nerve repair.

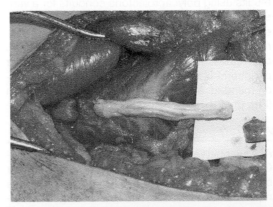

Fig. 8. Cable graft prepared on back table and held together with fibrin glue.

connectors can be placed around and secured to the cable ends. When the cable is brought to the surgical field it can efficiently be inset by securing both stumps into the cable graft/nerve connector construct (**Fig. 9**).

RESULTS

Many factors affecting outcomes are beyond the surgeon's control: patient age,[55] gap size,[56,57] level of injury,[58] and associated injuries.[59] One variable that can be controlled is timing of repair.[57]

A comprehensive literature review of clinical recovery following the major peripheral nerves of the upper extremities is hindered by the use of inconsistent outcome measurement tools, manipulated statistics, and author biases. Many studies report their results as successful, functional, or good. However, the surgeon's use of these terms may differ from the patient's. M3 (action against gravity) and S3 (pain and touch perception with 2-point discrimination greater than 15 mm) historically have been reported as functional. Based on this definition, Frykman and Gramyk[56] analyzed the available literature on grafted median, ulnar, and radial nerve repairs and estimated that useful motor recovery was obtained in 63% to 81% of cases and useful sensory recovery in 75% to 78% of cases. Others have reported similar outcomes ranges of 57% to 67% success following grafting of median[60] and ulnar nerves.[61] A more recent meta-analysis suggested that this minimal criterion of meaningful recovery could be achieved in around 60% of ulnar and median nerve repairs.[62]

When a stricter criterion of functional recovery is used (M4 and M5 and S3+ to S4) the results are disappointing. Reports suggest that sensory recovery to this level is achieved in only 50% of grafted median nerves[63,64] and 23% to 27% of grafted ulnar nerves.[64,65] A meta-analysis of 623 median or ulnar nerve injuries across 23 studies, found that S3+ or S4 sensory recovery was achieved 43% of the time, and M4 or 5 motor recovery 52% of the time. One exceptional study noted that long-term outcomes in high end-to-end radial nerve repairs achieved M4 to M5 strengths in 16 of 18 patients who returned for follow-up.[8]

Missile (bullet and shrapnel)-induced nerve injuries requiring repair portend a particularly dismal prognosis. Repair of 81 median nerves broken down by injury location resulted in successful outcomes in 69% of distal injuries, 33% of intermediate injuries, and 10% of proximal injuries. Concomitant ulnar nerve treatment resulted in no successful proximal repairs, 24% successful intermediate repairs, and 60% successful distal repairs.[66] Secer and colleagues,[58] reporting on similar injuries, found that only 15% of high, 30% of midlevel, and 50% of low ulnar nerve injuries achieved satisfactory results. In addition to large zones of nerve injury, this population has many concurrent non-nerve musculoskeletal injuries that compromise the end functional result. The disappointing outcomes following repair or reconstruction of major peripheral nerve injuries have led clinical investigators to search for alternative techniques, such as nerve transfers, which have potential to produce better outcomes.

SUMMARY

Although both the surgeon and the patient must maintain realistic expectations, appropriate diagnosis, timing of repair, and treatment strategies maximize the chances of a favorable outcome. I often tell my patients when counseling them for surgical repair, "Though there is a chance that the repair won't work, we certainly know what will happen if we do nothing." New repair and diagnostic tools will continue to refine the approach to this difficult problem.

REFERENCES

1. Chhabra A, Williams EH, Wang KC, et al. MR neurography of neuromas related to nerve injury and entrapment with surgical correlation. AJNR Am J Neuroradiol 2010;31(8):1363–8.

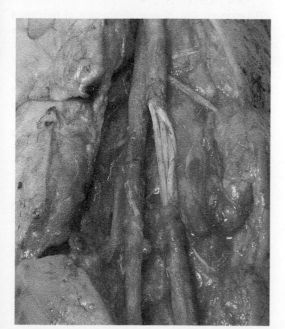

Fig. 9. Cable graft secured in place using nerve connectors.

2. Dahlin LB. Techniques of peripheral nerve repair. Scand J Surg 2008;97(4):310–6.

3. Liss AG, af Ekenstam FW, Wiberg M. Loss of neurons in the dorsal root ganglia after transection of a peripheral sensory nerve. An anatomical study in monkeys. Scand J Plast Reconstr Surg Hand Surg 1996;30(1):1–6.

4. Ma J, Novikov LN, Kellerth JO, et al. Early nerve repair after injury to the postganglionic plexus: an experimental study of sensory and motor neuronal survival in adult rats. Scand J Plast Reconstr Surg Hand Surg 2003;37(1):1–9.

5. Lundborg G, Rosen B. Hand function after nerve repair. Acta Physiol (Oxf) 2007;189(2):207–17.

6. Zachary LS, Dellon AL. Progression of the zone of injury in experimental nerve injuries. Microsurgery 1987;8(4):182–5.

7. Ring D, Chin K, Jupiter JB. Radial nerve palsy associated with high-energy humeral shaft fractures. J Hand Surg Am 2004;29(1):144–7.

8. Gurbuz Y, Kayalar M, Bal E, et al. Long-term functional results after radial nerve repair. Acta Orthop Traumatol Turc 2011;45(6):387–92.

9. Toros T, Karabay N, Ozaksar K, et al. Evaluation of peripheral nerves of the upper limb with ultrasonography: a comparison of ultrasonographic examination and the intra-operative findings. J Bone Joint Surg Br 2009;91(6):762–5.

10. Siemionow M, Brzezicki G. Chapter 8: Current techniques and concepts in peripheral nerve repair. Int Rev Neurobiol 2009;87:141–72.

11. Shao YC, Harwood P, Grotz MR, et al. Radial nerve palsy associated with fractures of the shaft of the humerus: a systematic review. J Bone Joint Surg Br 2005;87(12):1647–52.

12. Hamlin E Jr, Watkins AL. Regeneration in the ulnar, median and radial nerves. Surg Clin North Am 1947;27:1052–61.

13. Gulati AK. Restoration of denervated skeletal muscle transplants after reinnervation in rats. Restor Neurol Neurosci 1990;2(1):23–9.

14. Wiertz-Hoessels EL, Krediet P. Degeneration of the motor end-plates after neurectomy, in the rat and the rabbit. Acta Morphol Neerl Scand 1965;6:179–93.

15. Fu SY, Gordon T. Contributing factors to poor functional recovery after delayed nerve repair: prolonged axotomy. J Neurosci 1995;15(5 Pt 2):3876–85.

16. Tiel RL, Happel LT Jr, Kline DG. Nerve action potential recording method and equipment. Neurosurgery 1996;39(1):103–8 [discussion: 108–9].

17. Trumble TE, McCallister WV. Repair of peripheral nerve defects in the upper extremity. Hand Clin 2000;16(1):37–52.

18. Terzis J, Faibisoff B, Williams B. The nerve gap: suture under tension vs. graft. Plast Reconstr Surg 1975;56(2):166–70.

19. Yi C, Dahlin LB. Impaired nerve regeneration and Schwann cell activation after repair with tension. Neuroreport 2010;21(14):958–62.

20. Clark WL, Trumble TE, Swiontkowski MF, et al. Nerve tension and blood flow in a rat model of immediate and delayed repairs. J Hand Surg Am 1992;17(4):677–87.

21. Rydevik BL, Kwan MK, Myers RR, et al. An in vitro mechanical and histological study of acute stretching on rabbit tibial nerve. J Orthop Res 1990;8(5):694–701.

22. Brushart TM, Gerber J, Kessens P, et al. Contributions of pathway and neuron to preferential motor reinnervation. J Neurosci 1998;18(21):8674–81.

23. Robinson GA, Madison RD. Manipulations of the mouse femoral nerve influence the accuracy of pathway reinnervation by motor neurons. Exp Neurol 2005;192(1):39–45.

24. He YS, Zhong SZ. Acetylcholinesterase: a histochemical identification of motor and sensory fascicles in human peripheral nerve and its use during operation. Plast Reconstr Surg 1988;82(1):125–32.

25. Al-Qattan MM. Refinements in the technique of 'awake' electrical nerve stimulation in the management of chronic low ulnar nerve injuries. Injury 2004;35(11):1110–5.

26. Edshage S. Peripheral nerve suture. A technique for improved intraneural topography. Evaluation of some suture materials. Acta Chir Scand Suppl 1964;15(Suppl 331):1+.

27. Lundborg GA. 25-year perspective of peripheral nerve surgery: evolving neuroscientific concepts and clinical significance. J Hand Surg Am 2000;25(3):391–414.

28. Young L, Wray RC, Weeks PM. A randomized prospective comparison of fascicular and epineural digital nerve repairs. Plast Reconstr Surg 1981;68(1):89–93.

29. Chow JA, Van Beek AL, Bilos ZJ, et al. Anatomical basis for repair of ulnar and median nerves in the distal part of the forearm by group fascicular suture and nerve-grafting. J Bone Joint Surg Am 1986;68(2):273–80.

30. Palazzi S, Vila-Torres J, Lorenzo JC. Fibrin glue is a sealant and not a nerve barrier. J Reconstr Microsurg 1995;11(2):135–9.

31. Cruz NI, Debs N, Fiol RE. Evaluation of fibrin glue in rat sciatic nerve repairs. Plast Reconstr Surg 1986;78(3):369–73.

32. Isaacs JE, McDaniel CO, Owen JR, et al. Comparative analysis of biomechanical performance of available "nerve glues". J Hand Surg Am 2008;33(6):893–9.

33. Danielsen N, Varon S. Characterization of neurotrophic activity in the silicone-chamber model for nerve regeneration. J Reconstr Microsurg 1995; 11(3):231–5.

34. Ducic I, Fu R, Iorio ML. Innovative treatment of peripheral nerve injuries: combined reconstructive concepts. Ann Plast Surg 2012;68(2):180–7.

35. Evans PJ, Bain JR, Mackinnon SE, et al. Selective reinnervation: a comparison of recovery following microsuture and conduit nerve repair. Brain Res 1991;559(2):315–21.

36. Kokkalis ZT, Pu C, Small GA, et al. Assessment of processed porcine extracellular matrix as a protective barrier in a rabbit nerve wrap model. J Reconstr Microsurg 2011;27(1):19–28.

37. Williams LR, Longo FM, Powell HC, et al. Spatial-temporal progress of peripheral nerve regeneration within a silicone chamber: parameters for a bioassay. J Comp Neurol 1983;218(4):460–70.

38. Yang M, Rawson JL, Zhang EW, et al. Comparisons of outcomes from repair of median nerve and ulnar nerve defect with nerve graft and tubulization: a meta-analysis. J Reconstr Microsurg 2011;27(8): 451–60.

39. Braga-Silva J. The use of silicone tubing in the late repair of the median and ulnar nerves in the forearm. J Hand Surg Br 1999;24(6):703–6.

40. Stanec S, Stanec Z. Reconstruction of upper-extremity peripheral-nerve injuries with ePTFE conduits. J Reconstr Microsurg 1998;14(4):227–32.

41. Chiriac S, Facca S, Diaconu M, et al. Experience of using the bioresorbable copolyester poly(DL-lactide-epsilon-caprolactone) nerve conduit guide Neurolac for nerve repair in peripheral nerve defects: report on a series of 28 lesions. J Hand Surg Eur Vol 2012; 37(4):342–9.

42. Moore AM, Kasukurthi R, Magill CK, et al. Limitations of conduits in peripheral nerve repairs. Hand (N Y) 2009;4(2):180–6.

43. Krekoski CA, Neubauer D, Zuo J, et al. Axonal regeneration into acellular nerve grafts is enhanced by degradation of chondroitin sulfate proteoglycan. J Neurosci 2001;21(16):6206–13.

44. Hudson TW, Zawko S, Deister C, et al. Optimized acellular nerve graft is immunologically tolerated and supports regeneration. Tissue Eng 2004; 10(11–12):1641–51.

45. Neubauer D, Graham JB, Muir D. Chondroitinase treatment increases the effective length of acellular nerve grafts. Exp Neurol 2007;207(1):163–70.

46. Whitlock EL, Tuffaha SH, Luciano JP, et al. Processed allografts and type I collagen conduits for repair of peripheral nerve gaps. Muscle Nerve 2009;39(6):787–99.

47. Johnson PJ, Newton P, Hunter DA, et al. Nerve endoneurial microstructure facilitates uniform distribution of regenerative fibers: a post hoc comparison of midgraft nerve fiber densities. J Reconstr Microsurg 2011;27(2):83–90.

48. Giusti G, Willems WF, Kremer T, et al. Return of motor function after segmental nerve loss in a rat model: comparison of autogenous nerve graft, collagen conduit, and processed allograft (AxoGen). J Bone Joint Surg Am 2012;94(5):410–7.

49. Cho MS, Rinker BD, Weber RV, et al. Functional outcome following nerve repair in the upper extremity using processed nerve allograft. J Hand Surg Am 2012;37(11):2340–9.

50. Tang P, Kilic A, Konopka G, et al. Histologic and functional outcomes of nerve defects treated with acellular allograft versus cabled autograft in a rat model. Microsurgery Publication Pending.

51. Nichols CM, Brenner MJ, Fox IK, et al. Effects of motor versus sensory nerve grafts on peripheral nerve regeneration. Exp Neurol 2004;190(2): 347–55.

52. Moradzadeh A, Borschel GH, Luciano JP, et al. The impact of motor and sensory nerve architecture on nerve regeneration. Exp Neurol 2008; 212(2):370–6.

53. Isaacs J, Adams S, Mallu S, et al. Comparison of the performance of chronically versus freshly denervated autograft in nerve repair. J Hand Surg Am 2010;35(12):2001–7.

54. Meek MF, Coert JH, Robinson PH. Poor results after nerve grafting in the upper extremity: Quo vadis? Microsurgery 2005;25(5):396–402.

55. Lundborg G, Rosen B. Sensory relearning after nerve repair. Lancet 2001;358(9284):809–10.

56. Frykman G, Gramyk K. Results of nerve grafting. In: Gelberman R, editor. Operative nerve repair and reconstruction. Philadelphia: JB Lippincott; 1991. p. 553–68.

57. Ruijs AC, Jaquet JB, Kalmijn S, et al. Median and ulnar nerve injuries: a meta-analysis of predictors of motor and sensory recovery after modern microsurgical nerve repair. Plast Reconstr Surg 2005; 116(2):484–94 [discussion: 495–6].

58. Secer HI, Daneyemez M, Gonul E, et al. Surgical repair of ulnar nerve lesions caused by gunshot and shrapnel: results in 407 lesions. J Neurosurg 2007;107(4):776–83.

59. Galanakos SP, Zoubos AB, Ignatiadis I, et al. Repair of complete nerve lacerations at the forearm: an outcome study using Rosen-Lundborg protocol. Microsurgery 2011;31(4):253–62.

60. Kim DH, Kam AC, Chandika P, et al. Surgical management and outcomes in patients with median nerve lesions. J Neurosurg 2001;95(4):584–94.

61. Kim DH, Han K, Tiel RL, et al. Surgical outcomes of 654 ulnar nerve lesions. J Neurosurg 2003;98(5): 993–1004.

62. Brushart T. Nerve repair. New York: Oxford University Press; 2011.

63. Millesi H, Meissl G, Berger A. The interfascicular nerve-grafting of the median and ulnar nerves. J Bone Joint Surg Am 1972;54(4):727–50.

64. Millesi H, Meissl G, Berger A. Further experience with interfascicular grafting of the median, ulnar, and radial nerves. J Bone Joint Surg Am 1976; 58(2):209–18.

65. Moneim MS. Interfascicular nerve grafting. Clin Orthop Relat Res 1982;(163):65–74.

66. Roganovic Z. Missile-caused median nerve injuries: results of 81 repairs. Surg Neurol 2005; 63(5):410–8 [discussion: 418–9].

Evidence and Techniques in Rehabilitation Following Nerve Injuries

Christine B. Novak, PT, PhD[a,b,*],
Rebecca L. von der Heyde, PhD, OTR/L, CHT[c]

KEYWORDS

- Rehabilitation • Hand therapy • Treatment

KEY POINTS

- Rehabilitation is essential to optimize sensorimotor function and outcome following nerve injury.
- The strategies in early phase rehabilitation are related to pain and edema control, range of motion and neural mobility.
- Alterations in cortical mapping with nerve injury/recovery and sensory and motor reeducation support the importance of rehabilitation following nerve injury.

Injury to a peripheral nerve causes alterations in both the peripheral and central nervous system, and these changes begin immediately after injury and continue through recovery. These changes can result in substantial loss of motor and sensory function with high levels of impairment and a negative impact on health-related quality of life.[1,2] Following upper extremity peripheral nerve injury and surgery, rehabilitation is essential to optimize sensorimotor function and outcome. This review presents the evidence and related literature regarding a few key topics related to rehabilitation following peripheral nerve injury and surgery. In general, the level of evidence in the published literature is limited and comprises predominately low-level evidence.

GENERAL PRINCIPLES

In the early period following surgery, the main goals are related to range of motion, pain, and edema control. Patient education is important and begins preoperatively to ensure that patients understand nerve injury and recovery, the surgical procedure, and postoperative course.

The initial strategies following surgery include decreasing postoperative edema and pain management. Neuropathic pain has been associated with poor outcome and high levels of disability.[2–4] In cases of severe neuropathic pain, a multidisciplinary team approach may be necessary with referral to a pain management program. Immobilization following surgery is used to protect the nerve coaptation site. Initially, a bulky dressing is applied; in the authors' practice, this dressing is removed 2 to 3 days after surgery. Immobilization, such as a splint, sling, or shoulder immobilizer, is continued to protect the nerve coaptation site. Range of motion of the proximal and distal joints is encouraged to promote neural gliding. Similar to improved outcomes with tendon gliding and controlled motion following flexor tendon repair, the emphasis on controlled motion following nerve reconstruction has allowed the authors to incorporate early motion to decrease adhesions and promote neural gliding.

[a] Department of Surgery, University of Toronto, 399 Bathurst Street, EW2-422, Toronto, Ontario, M5T 2S8, Canada; [b] Toronto Rehab and Hand Program, University Health Network, 399 Bathurst Street, EW2-422, Toronto, Ontario, M5T 2S8, Canada; [c] Occupational Therapy Department, Concordia University Wisconsin, 12800 N Lake Shore Drive, Mequon, WI 53097, USA
* Corresponding author. TWH Hand Centre, 399 Bathurst Street, EW2-422, Toronto, Ontario M5T 2S8, Canada.
E-mail address: Christine.novak@uhn.ca

Hand Clin 29 (2013) 383–392
http://dx.doi.org/10.1016/j.hcl.2013.04.012
0749-0712/13/$ – see front matter © 2013 Elsevier Inc. All rights reserved.

In the literature, there are varying reports on the recommended period of immobilization following nerve repair or graft and vary between a few days to several weeks. In part, this variability depends on the tension applied to the repair site with range of motion, patient factors, and surgeon preference.[5–10] Early postoperative range of motion is advocated with the hypothesis that this motion will minimize scarring and encourage neural mobility. Longer periods of immobilization are based on the hypothesis that early range of motion will increase scar and collagen formation at the nerve coaptation site and, thus, impede nerve regeneration.[5–9,11–15] The ideal period of time for immobilization to balance protection of the nerve coaptation site and to promote neural mobility remains to be established. For repair sites that may undergo tension with movement, such as with a direct end-to-end repair, this period may be as long as 3 weeks, particularly if the joint range of motion induces increased tension on the nerve. For nerve graft or transfer whereby no tension is transferred to the coaptation site with movement, the time of immobilization or protected motion may be shortened to 3 to 10 days following surgery, although some surgeons continue restriction of movement for 3 weeks.

The period of immobilization is also dependent on the surrounding soft tissues, which may have been repaired during the surgical procedure. In cases of brachial plexus reconstruction whereby the pectoralis major is detached and reattached, a 4-week period of immobilization in adduction and internal rotation of the shoulder is recommended. Range of motion of the proximal and distal joints that is not included in the immobilization will promote neural mobility and gliding and assist in both pain and edema control. Following immobilization, range-of-motion exercises should continue until full range of motion is achieved. As muscle reinnervation occurs, patients should be reevaluated frequently to ensure full range of motion is maintained and monitored for muscle reinnervation. Muscle imbalance may be persistent until sufficient strength is attained and normal movement patterns can be performed.

MOTOR NERVE TRANSFER

Nerve transfers present the unique situation whereby a muscle is innervated by a new proximal nerve source, thus, altering the previously established cortical map and motor patterns. Therefore, rehabilitation strategies following nerve transfer must be directed to the sensorimotor systems via increased emphasis on cortical remapping and movement patterns, in addition to increased muscle strength and muscle balance. Motor nerve transfers have been more commonly used as a salvage procedure when nerve repair or graft was not possible, such as an intercostal to musculocutaneous nerve transfer in brachial plexus avulsion injuries.[16–18] Although reinnervation of the biceps muscle was successful with adequate elbow flexion, the overall patient outcome was less than optimal because of the devastating nature of the injury and no recovery of hand function. More recently, the use of nerve transfers has expanded to include more distal nerve injury as well as spinal cord injury; outcomes with these nerve transfers have been encouraging.[10,19–24]

Numerous clinical studies have reported outcomes following nerve transfer, including patients with nerve injuries to the brachial plexus, median, ulnar, and radial nerves.[10,19–24] Comparison between surgical procedures and studies is challenging because of the wide variety of preoperative and postoperative outcome assessments, including patient self-report and surgeon or therapist assessment. Garg and colleagues[25] performed a systematic literature review to evaluate the outcomes following nerve transfer or nerve graft in patients with upper brachial plexus injuries. Using the British Medical Research Council (MRC) muscle grading system, the investigators report improved outcomes in shoulder and elbow function following nerve transfer. However, it is important to recognize that not all studies use the MRC scale uniformly.

In the authors' literature review, they did not find any studies that specifically evaluated the efficacy of rehabilitation following nerve transfers. In most outcome studies, the nerve transfer surgical technique and postoperative rehabilitation are described in the methodology and outcomes are reported for the procedure, including postoperative management. The authors' treatment of patients with motor nerve transfer includes preoperative education and postoperatively early and late-phase rehabilitation.

With evidence of muscle reinnervation, rehabilitation is focused on sensorimotor reeducation and restoration of muscle balance. Because a new donor nerve is transferred to the recipient nerve to target muscle reinnervation, the motor patterns and cortical mapping are altered. Initially, contraction of the reinnervated muscle will require contraction of the donor muscle; with the establishment of new motor patterns and cortical remapping, the action will be performed without the donor muscle. As with any new task, practice and repetition with appropriate feedback is necessary to achieve success and correct motor patterns.[26]

DIGITAL NERVE REPAIR

The literature pertaining to rehabilitation following nerve repair attends primarily to the major peripheral nerves of the upper extremity, offering evidence for both conservative and postoperative management of median, radial, and ulnar injuries. A dearth of information regarding therapeutic interventions and expectations following digital nerve repair is noted despite progress in surgical techniques. Therefore, this section reviews the current literature on digital nerve repair as a means to direct therapeutic decision making and offer evidence-based benchmarks for clinical outcomes.

Recovery Based on Surgical Procedure

From a rehabilitative perspective, knowledge of the type of repair or reconstruction offers the therapist insight to potential outcomes, including time frames for sensory recovery. Repair following digital nerve injury is typically accomplished using one of 4 techniques: end-to-end neurorrhaphy, nerve grafts, nerve conduits, or end-to-side neurorrhaphy.[27] Lohmeyer and colleagues[28] reported that direct repair is used in approximately 82% of cases, whereas the use of a graft or conduit is optimal about 18% of the time.

Studies have used a combination of subjective and objective measures as a means to assess outcomes following digital nerve repair. Most common are static/moving 2-point discrimination and pain.[29] Static 2-point discrimination is reported both in millimeters and using the modified guidelines of the American Society for Surgery of the Hand.[29] Less often, researchers have included sensory threshold testing; range of motion; and more recently, self-report measures, such as the Disabilities of the Arm, Shoulder, and Hand (DASH), the Michigan Hand Outcomes Questionnaire (MHQ), and the Cold Intolerance Severity Score (CISS).[2–4,30–42]

Examples of sensory recovery as reported in static 2-point discrimination can be gleaned from current research.[28,43–47] These studies include current approaches of nerve conduit and grafting techniques with follow-up measurement ranging from 6 months to 4 years. Of particular note are the favorable outcomes of decellularized nerve allografts at the 9-month time frame with static 2-point discrimination of 5.5 mm.[46] More typically, at 1 year after surgery, patients with conduits and vein grafts were noted to have results at or near 7 mm.[28,43,47] Wang and colleagues[48] evaluated 74 patients following primary digital nerve repair (at least 1 year after surgery) for comparison, and 49% of patients had static 2-point discrimination of 7 mm or less. A recent systematic review including 14 articles with data for 191 nerves found no statistically significant difference in outcomes between differing digital nerve repair techniques.[27] This review included a mean follow-up of 28 months and reported only 25% of patients having excellent results (<6 mm).

Variables that have been associated with outcomes following digital nerve repair include age, length of follow-up after surgery, delay in repair from time of the initial injury, type of trauma, and gap length. Of these variables, younger age has been established as a significant predictor of recovery after digital nerve repair by multiple investigators.[27,48,49] Weinzweig and colleagues[49] also identified mechanism of injury as a variable of significance, whereas Rinker and Liau[44] reported that smokers and patients with workers' compensation demonstrated worse sensory recovery at 12 months. These studies from the surgical literature provide data for comparison of patient outcomes over time.

Immobilization Following Repair

Historically, patients with a digital nerve repair have been treated with immobilization of the proximal interphalangeal (PIP) joint at 30° of flexion for 3 weeks following surgery. Although some surgeons have progressed from this conservative approach, the strategy of blocking the PIP joint to avoid deleterious tension at the repair site remains in practice. The primary concern in using this approach is the likelihood of persistent flexion contractures at the PIP joint that require additional time and interventions to resolve. The close-packed position of the PIP joint is full extension, affording maximal length of the connective tissue structures surrounding the joint, optimal articulation of the joint surfaces, and minimal excess space within the joint. Any positioning toward flexion at the PIP negatively impacts these variables, allowing volar plate compression and contraction of the checkrein ligaments.[50] Digital nerves repaired with tension in extension may require immobilization in a shortened position; however, the amount of flexion and progression of active extension should be pursued on a case-by-case basis.

Positioning of joints after digital nerve repair as discussed in the current, surgical literature is directed toward the metacarpophalangeal (MP) joint. In a cadaveric study that measured the tension produced during passive finger range of motion, there was no appreciable tension with PIP motion regardless of MP position within the normal range.[51] However, when the MP joint was passively moved into hyperextension, tension on the nerve was notably increased ($\sim$4N). The investigators recommended the use of orthotics to block the MP joint in flexion to avoid tension of the digital nerve. Chen and colleagues[43,45] also reported on this type of MP blocking orthotic.[43,45] Primarily intending to assess the outcomes of a dorsal digital nerve island flap and a proper digital nerve dorsal branch transfer, the investigators used a position of 70° MP flexion and 0° PIP and distal interphalangeal extension for immobilization following surgery.[43,45] The results of both studies yielded the return of sensibility commensurate with similar studies.

The combined injury of flexor tendons and digital nerves in zone II provides a typical case in which PIP flexion is used postsurgically. To address this specific diagnosis, Yu and colleagues[52] compared patients with primary, isolated digital nerve repairs to those with a concomitant flexor tendon repair. No significant differences were observed between groups in 2-point discrimination or sensory threshold despite the tendon/nerve group being mobilized using a Kleinert protocol starting at day 4 and the nerve group being immobilized for 21 days. The investigators concluded that immobilization of digital nerves for 3 weeks was unnecessary if tension on the healing nerve could be avoided. It is of note that the Kleinert protocol includes a dorsal blocking orthosis with MP flexion and interphalangeal extension as referenced in previous studies.[43,45,51]

ELECTRICAL STIMULATION

As an adjunct to rehabilitation, a variety of modalities have been recommended for treatment following nerve injury and repair. A commonly used modality is electrical muscle stimulation; it has also been reported as electrical stimulation, neuromuscular electrical stimulation, functional electrical stimulation, and transcutaneous electrical stimulation. The parameters of the electrical stimulation vary with different types of applications, and there are different protocols described in the rehabilitation literature.[53] For stimulation of denervated muscle, a direct current or galvanic stimulation is used; for innervated muscle, an indirect current may be used. In general, the level of evidence in clinical studies for electrical stimulation of denervated muscle is limited and largely based on small series reports.

Following injury to a motor nerve, a cascade of events occurs resulting in muscle denervation with both structural and functional changes to the muscle.[54] Short-term denervation atrophy is reversible and does not result in long-term deficits. However, long-term denervation atrophy results in irreversible pathologic changes to the muscle. Following denervation, the optimal outcome occurs when motor axons are promptly supplied to denervated muscle, thus, providing rapid reinnervation. Longer durations of denervation are associated with poorer outcomes. However, the definitive timeline to muscle reinnervation before irreversible changes remains undefined but is likely in the period of 18 to 24 months; muscle reinnervation is possible for longer periods following injury with incontinuity nerve lesions compared with transection injuries. Overall, the evidence in the literature supports the assertion that the best recovery of muscle function occurs with shorter durations of muscle denervation.

The treatment goals remain focused on providing innervation to the denervated muscle before irreversible muscle changes associated with denervation. Rehabilitation strategies for the treatment of denervated muscle have included electrical stimulation with the goal of prolonging the time before muscle degeneration by providing an external source of stimulation to the muscle fibers. Studies of both innervated and denervated muscle have shown benefits to the contractile properties of the muscle with increased contractile activity, which may be induced through electrical stimulation.[55] However, in cases of denervated muscle, the efficacy of electrical stimulation to prolong the time period before irreversible muscle atrophy and increase the capacity for reinnervation remains unanswered. In a rat sciatic nerve model, improved functional recovery was reported for low-intensity stimulation.[56] However, at higher intensities (2 Hz), adverse effects (impaired functional recovery) of electrical stimulation were reported.[56] Although these adverse effects may not be directly transferred to humans, it does raise the question of the benefit versus detrimental effects that may be attributed to electrical stimulation. There are many clinical reports using electrical stimulation following motor nerve injury, and there are a limited number of published clinical studies that have provided very low levels of evidence. Many of the studies using nerve injury animal models used direct electrical stimulation with implanted intramuscular wires, and some studies used implanted stimulators. Typically in clinical practice, a direct current using galvanic stimulation is applied via surface electrodes. The authors' literature review did not reveal any efficacy trials in humans to support the use of direct current electrical stimulation with external electrodes and improvement of outcomes in denervated muscle, specifically to prolong the time for muscle innervation. Given the lack of strong clinical evidence and the variation of the technique to apply the electrical stimulation in the clinical setting of patients with nerve injury, the authors do not advocate the use of galvanic stimulation in denervated muscle.

Electrical stimulation following motor nerve injury is typically applied directly to the muscle with the goal of modifying the muscle fibers. Other approaches to optimize muscle recovery have been directed toward enhancing nerve regeneration and decreasing the duration of denervation. These strategies have included the use of electrical stimulation, nerve growth factors, conditioning lesions, and immunosuppressive drugs. The electrical stimulation used in this type of application is targeted to the nerve with the goal of accelerating nerve regeneration and, thus, providing more timely muscle reinnervation and decreasing the time of muscle denervation. Studies investigating 1 hour of electrical stimulation in rodent and rabbit models have shown beneficial effects with accelerated reinnervation and functional recovery.[57,58] In a clinical study, Gordon and colleagues[59] investigated patients with carpal tunnel syndrome who were treated for 1 hour with electrical stimulation of the median nerve immediately after carpal tunnel release. Postoperative low frequency electrical stimulation of the nerve was associated with accelerated axonal regeneration and improved motor and sensory parameters. These studies provide proof of principle for the use of low-frequency electrical stimulation and accelerated nerve regeneration.

Electrical stimulation of innervated muscle may provide increased strength, which is necessary for function; but muscle strength is only one component of upper extremity motor function. The establishment of good motor function following nerve injury also requires the restoration of full passive joint range of motion, muscle balance, and normal motor patterns. During the period of time from nerve injury to reinnervation, many patients develop altered compensatory movement patterns, muscle weakness from disuse rather than denervation, and altered sensorimotor cortical mapping. Integration and coordination of motor and sensory reeducation are necessary to optimize outcome.

SENSORY REEDUCATION

Following nerve injury, in addition to the peripheral changes that occur at the muscle and sensory end-organ level, there are rapid changes that occur in the cortex. Injury to a sensory nerve will result in decreased sensory input to the cortex and reorganization of the somatosensory cortical map.[60–63] Rehabilitation treatments have been focused on strategies to alter the detrimental effects of deafferentation. Following several clinical reports in the literature in the 1970s,[29,64–66] sensory reeducation has been routinely used after peripheral nerve injury to optimize outcomes. Numerous clinical studies have reported outcomes after median, ulnar, and digital nerve injuries and repair with descriptions of postoperative sensory reeducation.[64,66–69] Recent reviews have evaluated the literature related to outcomes following sensory reeducation in patients with upper extremity nerve repair.[70,71] In general, there is evidence to support the use of sensory reeducation following peripheral nerve injury and repair. However, the limitations of the studies reviewed included the use of a variety of reported outcome measures and the lack of detailed descriptions for the sensory reeducation programs used.

Sensory reeducation is used to improve sensibility and also to decrease pain, allodynia, and hyperalgesia. A variety of techniques have been described, including varying textures, localization and discrimination, and mobility tasks. As sensibility improves, the strategies are increased to challenge the sensory system and optimize cortical remapping and normal movement patterns.

Sensory reeducation programs typically begin with evidence of sensory end-organ reinnervation. Early phase reeducation programs before reinnervation have been described to enhance the sensory cortex remapping.[69,72–74] These techniques have included mirror imagery, temporary anesthesia, and audio-tactile and visuo-tactile training.

SELF-REPORT OUTCOMES ASSESSMENT

The use of outcome measures to assess and demonstrate patient progress has recently changed from a preference to an expectation. A myriad of patient self-report outcome measures are available for use by the hand surgeon and therapist ranging from general to regional to disease-specific. The following section aims to summarize both well-established and more novel tools that are being used to evaluate outcomes in patients with peripheral nerve injuries.

DASH

The most widely used regional, upper extremity self-report outcome measure for disability, the DASH, was designed to allow comparison of conditions throughout the upper extremity while considering it a single functional unit.[34] Two concepts of symptoms and functional status compose the 30-item tool and are assessed from 1 (no difficulty, symptoms, or limitations) to 5 (unable to complete activities and extreme symptoms and signs). Scores range from 0 to 100, with higher scores indicating increased perceived disability. Continued testing by the original investigators yielded a suggested minimal detectable change (MDC) score of 12.75, with a suggested mean MDC of 13 (range 8–17) published on the DASH website (http://www.dash.iwh.on.ca/faq).[30]

Specific to nerve injuries, the DASH has been suggested as a responsive tool for use with patients following carpal tunnel release.[33,36] Commonly used in clinical research, this tool has also been used to identify predictors of disability in patients with peripheral nerve injuries. Studies by Novak and colleagues[1,2] found significantly higher perceived disability in patients with brachial plexus injuries, with mean DASH scores ranging from 44 to 52. The nerve injured, pain, and older age were distinguished as predictors of higher DASH scores in addition to work status, time since injury, cold sensitivity, and pain catastrophizing.[1,2]

MHQ

The MHQ consists of 67 questions that address domains of overall hand function, physical function with activities of daily living tasks, esthetics, and satisfaction with hand function.[40] Questions are formatted in Likert scales ranging from 1 to 5; summed and averaged scores are normalized from 0 to 100. The MHQ is defined as hand specific; it addresses the function of each upper extremity as a means of analyzing independent use, hand dominance, and bilateral involvement.[39]

Relative to peripheral nerve outcomes, the MHQ has been found to be sensitive to clinical change for patients with carpal tunnel syndrome and after carpal tunnel release.[36,42,75] Minimally clinically important differences have been published specifically for patients with carpal tunnel syndrome as pain, 23; function, 13; and work, 8.[76] In addition, this tool was suggested to have a higher overall responsiveness as compared with the DASH and Patient-Specific Functional Scale (PSFS) in a sample of 81 patients with carpal tunnel, wrist pain, and finger contractures.[36] The Brief MHQ was recently introduced to complete when a shorter time is desirable.[77]

Disease-Specific Measure: the Boston Questionnaire for Carpal Tunnel Syndrome

The Boston Questionnaire was developed as a disease-specific measure for clients with carpal tunnel syndrome, including an 11-item Symptom Severity Scale and an 8-item Functional Status Scale.[78] Items are evaluated for a typical day in the past 2 weeks and answered on a Likert scale. A score of 1 indicates a low level of symptom/difficulty, whereas a score of 5 indicates that patients are highly symptomatic or unable to complete functional tasks. The answers are averaged, with higher scores indicating decreased status. The Boston Questionnaire has been shown to be reliable, valid, and sensitive to change in clients with carpal tunnel syndrome[78–83] and more sensitive to clinical change than generic[33,75,79,84] and regional measures.[75] Disease-specific self-report measures allow inclusion of specific items related to the condition or diagnosis of interest.

CISS

The CISS is a 6-item questionnaire developed to assess the impact of cold intolerance on daily function.[35] Using Likert scales, patients are asked to determine cold-induced symptom type, incidence, relief, and prevention. In addition, 2 questions regarding functional tasks that provoke symptoms and those that are limited because of symptoms are included in the tool. The total score ranges from 0 to 100, with higher scores indicating greater cold intolerance. The CISS has been reported as reliable and valid for patients with upper extremity injuries.[31,32,35,38,85] Specific to nerve injury, a study of 61 patients with brachial plexus injuries yielded a mean CISS score of 34 that was significantly higher in women.[86] Pain ratings, perceived disability, and time since injury were identified as predictors of cold intolerance in the study.

PSFS

The PSFS is a self-report measure that asks patients to independently identify specific activities that they have difficulty with or are unable to perform.[87] The tool incorporates 10-cm visual analog scales that are anchored based on the perceived ability for up to 5 separate activities. The PSFS was confirmed to have construct and concurrent validity, good reliability, and responsiveness for patients with upper extremity musculoskeletal problems.[36,88] A minimal detectable change of 3 with a minimally important difference of 1.2 was reported. Specific to nerve injury, the PSFS was found to be sensitive to change for patients with carpal tunnel syndrome up to 6 months after surgery, and construct validity was confirmed in a sample of 157 patients with upper extremity nerve injury.[36,89] Patients in the latter study had a mean PSFS score of 3.1; significantly lower scores were reported in those with brachial plexus injuries. The PSFS provides the opportunity for patients to select items that are specifically relevant. However, comparison between patients is more challenging because of the variation in activities selected. The use of more generic questionnaires, such as the

DASH and MHQ, in combination with the PSFS may provide a more comprehensive evaluation.

SUMMARY

The strategies used in rehabilitation following peripheral nerve injury and reconstruction is supported in basic science and small cohort clinical studies. Although strong evidence with randomized controlled clinical trials is lacking, the strategies related to early mobilization, altered cortical mapping and remapping, and sensory and motor reeducation support the importance of rehabilitation following nerve injury. Future studies using valid, reliable outcome measures (quantitative, qualitative, and self-reported) will provide additional direct evidence for the use of postoperative rehabilitation to optimize recovery and minimize disability.

REFERENCES

1. Novak CB, Anastakis DJ, Beaton DE, et al. Patient reported outcome following peripheral nerve injury. J Hand Surg Am 2009;34:281-7.

2. Novak CB, Anastakis DJ, Beaton DE, et al. Biomedical and psychosocial factors associated with disability after peripheral nerve injury. J Bone Joint Surg Am 2011;93:929-36.

3. Jensen MP, Chodroff MJ, Dworkin RH. The impact of neuropathic pain on health-related quality of life: review and implications. Neurology 2007;68: 1178-82.

4. Novak CB, Katz J. Neuropathic pain in patients with upper extremity nerve injury. Physiother Can 2010;62:190-201.

5. Birch R. Nerve repair. In: Wolfe SW, Hotchkiss RN, Pederson WC, et al, editors. Green's operative hand surgery. Philadelphia: Elsevier Churchill Livingstone; 2011. p. 1035-74.

6. Boyd KU, Fox IK, Mackinnon SE. Nerve transfers. In: Neligan PC, Chang J, editors. Plastic surgery hand and upper extremity. London: Elsevier Saunders; 2013. p. 719-44.

7. Farnedo S, Thorfinn J, Dahlin LB. Peripheral nerve injuries of the upper extremity. In: Neligan PC, Chang J, editors. Plastic surgery hand and upper extremity. London: Elsevier Saunders; 2013. p. 694-718.

8. Lundborg G. Nerve injury and repair. Philadelphia: Elsevier Churchill Livingstone; 2005.

9. Mackinnon SE, Dellon AL. Surgery of the peripheral nerve. New York: Thieme Medical Publishers; 1988.

10. Mackinnon SE, Novak CB. Nerve transfers. Hand Clin 1999;15:643-66.

11. Millesi H. Factors affecting the outcome of peripheral nerve surgery. Microsurgery 2006;26: 295-302.

12. Lee WP, Constantinescu MA, Butler PE. Effect of early mobilization on healing of nerve repair: histologic observations in a canine model. Plast Reconstr Surg 1999;104:1718-25.

13. Millesi H, Zoch G, Rath T. The gliding apparatus of peripheral nerve and its clinical significance. Ann Hand Surg 1990;9:87-97.

14. Millesi H, Zoch G, Reihsner R. Mechanical properties of peripheral nerves. Clin Orthop Relat Res 1995;314:76-83.

15. Schmidhammer R, ZZandieh S, Hopf R, et al. Alleviated tension at the repair site enhances functional regeneration: the effect of full range of motion mobilization on the regeneration of peripheral nerves - histologic, electrophysiologic and functional results in a rat model. J Trauma 2004;56: 571-84.

16. Chuang DC, Yeh MC, Wei FC. Intercostal nerve transfer of the musculocutaneous nerve in avulsed brachial plexus injuries: evaluation of 66 patients. J Hand Surg Am 1992;17:822-8.

17. Chuang DC, Epstein MD, Yeh MC, et al. Functional restoration of elbow flexion in brachial plexus injuries: results in 167 patients. J Hand Surg 1993; 18:285-91.

18. Waikakul S, Wongtragul S, Vanadurongwan V. Restoration of elbow flexion in avulsion brachial plexus injury: comparing spinal accessory intercostal nerve neurotization. J Hand Surg 1999;24: 571-7.

19. Lurje A. Concerning surgical treatment of traumatic injury of the upper division of the brachial plexus (Erb's type). Ann Surg 1948;127:317-26.

20. Mackinnon SE, Novak CB, Myckatyn TM, et al. Results of reinnervation of the biceps and brachialis muscles with a double fascicular transfer. J Hand Surg Am 2005;30:978-85.

21. Novak CB, Mackinnon SE. A distal anterior interosseous nerve transfer to the deep motor branch of the ulnar nerve for reconstruction of high ulnar nerve injuries. J Reconstr Microsurg 2002;18: 459-63.

22. Novak CB, Tung TH, Mackinnon SE. Patient outcome following a thoracodorsal to musculocutaneous nerve transfer for reconstruction of elbow flexion. Br J Plast Surg 2003;55:416-9.

23. Oberlin C, Beal D, Leechavengvongs S, et al. Nerve transfer to biceps muscle using a part of ulnar nerve for C5-C6 avulsion of the brachial plexus: anatomical study and report of four cases. J Hand Surg Am 1994;19:232-7.

24. Tung TH, Novak CB, Mackinnon SE. Nerve transfers to the biceps and brachialis branches to improve elbow flexion strength after brachial plexus injuries. J Neurosurg 2003;98:313-8.

25. Garg R, Merrell GA, Hillstrom HJ, et al. Comparison of nerve transfers and nerve grafting for

traumatic upper plexus palsy: a systematic review and analysis. J Bone Joint Surg Am 2011; 93:819–29.

26. Duff SV. Impact of peripheral nerve injury on sensorimotor control. J Hand Ther 2005;18:277–91.

27. Mermans JF, Franssen BB, Serroyen J, et al. Digital nerve injuries: a review of predictors of sensory recovery after microsurgical digital nerve repair. Hand 2012;7:233–41.

28. Lohmeyer JA, Siemers F, Machens HG, et al. The clinical use of artificial nerve conduits for digital nerve repair: a prospective cohort study and literature review. J Reconstr Microsurg 2009;25:55–61.

29. Dellon AL, Kallman CH. Evaluation of functional sensation in the hand. J Hand Surg Am 1983;8: 865–70.

30. Beaton DE, Katz JN, Fossel AH, et al. Measuring the whole or the parts? Validity, reliability and responsiveness of the Disabilities of the Arm, Shoulder and Hand outcome measure in different regions of the upper extremity. J Hand Ther 2001; 14:128–46.

31. Carlsson I, Cederlund R, Hoglund P, et al. Hand injuries and cold sensitivity: reliability and validity of cold sensitivity questionnaires. Disabil Rehabil 2008;30:1920–8.

32. Carlsson I, Rosen B, Dahlin LB. Self-reported cold sensitivity in normal subjects and in patients with traumatic hand injuries or hand-arm vibration syndrome. BMC Musculoskelet Disord 2010;11: 89–99.

33. Gay RE, Amadio PC, Johnson JC. Comparative responsiveness of the Disabilities of the Arm, Shoulder and Hand, the Carpal Tunnel Questionnaire, and the SF-36 to clinical change after carpal tunnel release. J Hand Surg Am 2003;28:250–4.

34. Hudak PL, Amadio PC, Bombardier C. Development of an upper extremity outcome measure: the DASH (Disabilities of the Arm, Shoulder and Hand). Am J Ind Med 1996;29:602–8.

35. Irwin MS, Gilbert SE, Terenghi G, et al. Cold intolerance following peripheral nerve injury. Natural history and factors predicting severity of symptoms. J Hand Surg Am 1997;22:308–16.

36. McMillan CR, Binhammer PA. Which outcome measure is the best? Evaluating responsiveness of the Disabilities of the Arm, Shoulder and Hand questionnaire, the Michigan Hand Questionnaire and the Patient-Specific Functional Scale following hand and wrist surgery. Hand 2009;4:311–8.

37. Ruijs AC, Jaquet JB, Kalmijn S, et al. Median and ulnar nerve injuries: a meta-analysis of predictors of motor and sensory recovery after modern microsurgical nerve repair. Plast Reconstr Surg 2005; 116:484–94.

38. Ruijs AC, Jaquet JB, Daanen HA, et al. Cold intolerance of the hand measured by the CISS questionnaire in the normative study population. J Hand Surg Am 2006;31:533–6.

39. Amadio PC. Outcome assessment in hand surgery and hand therapy: an update. J Hand Ther 2001; 14:63–8.

40. Chung KC, Pillsbury MS, Walters MR, et al. Reliability and validity testing of the Michigan Hand Outcomes Questionnaire. J Hand Surg Am 1998; 23:575–87.

41. Chung KC, Hamill JB, Walters MR, et al. The Michigan Hand Outcomes Questionnaire (MHQ): assessment of responsiveness to clinical change. Ann Plast Surg 1999;42:619–22.

42. Kotsis SV, Chung KC, Arbor A. Responsiveness of the Michigan Hand Outcomes Questionnaire and the Disabilities of the Arm, Shoulder and Hand Questionnaire in carpal tunnel surgery. J Hand Surg Am 2005;30:81–6.

43. Chen C, Zhang X, Shao X, et al. Treatment of a combination of volar soft tissue and proper digital nerve defects using the dorsal digital nerve island flap. J Hand Surg Am 2010;35:1655–62.

44. Rinker B, Liau JY. A prospective study comparing woven polyglycolic acid and autogenous vein conduits for reconstruction of digital nerve gaps. J Hand Surg Am 2011;36:775–8.

45. Chen C, Tang P, Zhang X. Finger sensory reconstruction with transfer of the proper digital nerve dorsal branch. J Hand Surg Am 2013;38: 82–9.

46. Karabekmez FE, Duymaz A, Moran SL. Early clinical outcomes with the use of decellularized nerve allograft for repair of sensory defects within the hand. Hand 2009;4:245–9.

47. Bushnell BD, McWilliams AD, Whitener GB, et al. Early clinical experience with collagen nerve tubes in digital nerve repair. J Hand Surg Am 2008;33: 1081–7.

48. Wang W, Crain GM, Baylis W, et al. Outcome of digital nerve injuries in adults. J Hand Surg Am 1996; 21:138–43.

49. Weinzweig N, Chin G, Mead M, et al. Recovery of sensibility after digital neurorraphy: a clinical investigation of prognostic factors. Ann Plast Surg 2000; 44:610–7.

50. Hammert WC. Hand fractures and joint injuries. In: Neligan PC, Chang J, editors. Plastic surgery: hand and upper extremity. St Louis (MO): Elsevier Saunders; 2013. p. 138–60.

51. Goldberg SH, Jobin CM, Hayes AG, et al. Biomechanics and histology of intact and repaired digital nerves: an in vitro study. J Hand Surg Am 2007;32: 474–82.

52. Yu RS, Catalano LW, Barron OA, et al. Limited, protected postsurgical motion does not affect the results of digital nerve repair. J Hand Surg Am 2004;29:302–6.

53. Michlovitz SL. Is there a role for ultrasound and electrical stimulation following injury to tendon and nerve? J Hand Ther 2005;18:292–6.

54. Lien SC, Cederna PS, Kuzon WM. Optimizing skeletal muscle reinnervation with nerve transfer. Hand Clin 2008;24:445–54.

55. Dow DE, Cederna PS, Hassett CA, et al. Number of contractions to maintain mass and force of a denervated rat muscle. Muscle Nerve 2004;30:77–86.

56. Lu MC, Tsai CC, Chen SC, et al. Use of electrical stimulation at different current levels to promote recovery after peripheral nerve injury in rats. J Trauma 2009;67:1066–72.

57. Ahlborn P, Schachner M, Irintchev A. One hour electrical stimulation accelerates functional recovery after femoral nerve repair. Exp Neurol 2007;208:137–44.

58. Gordon T, Chan KM, Sulaiman OA, et al. Accelerating axon growth to overcome limitations in functional recovery after peripheral nerve injury. Neurosurgery 2009;65:132–44.

59. Gordon T, Amirjani N, Edwards DC, et al. Brief post-surgical electrical stimulation accelerates axon regeneration and muscle reinnervation without affecting the functional measures in carpal tunnel syndrome patients. Exp Neurol 2010;223:192–202.

60. Merzenich MM, Harrington T. The sense of flutter-vibration evoked by stimulation of the hairy skin of primates: comparison of human sensory capacity with the responses of mechanoreceptive afferents innervating the hairy skin of monkeys. Exp Brain Res 1969;9:236–60.

61. Merzenich MM, Jenkins WM. Reorganization of cortical representations of the hand following alterations of skin inputs induced by nerve injury, skin island transfers and experience. J Hand Ther 1993;6:89–104.

62. Wall JT, Kaas JH, Sur M, et al. Functional reorganization in somatosensory cortical areas 3b and 1 of adult monkeys after median nerve repair: possible relationships to sensory recovery in humans. J Neurosci 1986;6:218–33.

63. Wall JT, Kaas JH. Long-term cortical consequences of reinnervation errors after nerve regeneration in monkeys. Brain Res 1986;372:400–4.

64. Dellon AL, Curtis RM, Edgerton MT. Reeducation of sensation in the hand after nerve injury and repair. Plast Reconstr Surg 1974;53:297–305.

65. Wynn Parry CB. Rehabilitation of the hand. London: Butterworth; 1958.

66. Wynn Parry CB, Salter M. Sensory reeducation after median nerve lesions. Hand 1976;10:63–7.

67. Imai H, Tajima T, Natsumi Y. Successful reeducation of functional sensibility after median nerve repair at the wrist. J Hand Surg Am 1991;16:60–5.

68. Novak CB, Kelly L, Mackinnon SE. Sensory recovery after median nerve grafting. J Hand Surg Am 1992;17:59–68.

69. Rosen B, Lundborg G. Sensory re-education following nerve repair. In: Slutsky DJ, editor. Upper extremity nerve repair - tips and techniques: a Master Skills Publication. Rosemont (VA): American Society for Surgery of the Hand; 2008. p. 159–78.

70. Miller LK, Chester R, Jerosch-Herold C. Effects of sensory reeducation programs on functional hand sensibility after median and ulnar repair: a systematic review. J Hand Ther 2012;25:297–307.

71. Oud T, Beelen A, Eijffinger E, et al. Sensory re-education after nerve injury of the upper limb: a systematic review. Clin Rehabil 2007;21:483–94.

72. Rosen B, Lundborg G. Training with a mirror in rehabilitation of the hand. Scand J Plast Reconstr Surg Hand Surg 2005;39:104–8.

73. Lundborg G, Rosen B, Lindberg S. Hearing as substitution for sensation: a new principle for artificial sensibility. J Hand Surg Am 1999;24:219–24.

74. Rosen B, Bjorkman A, Lundborg G. Improved sensory relearning after nerve repair induced by selective temporary anaesthesia - a new concept in hand rehabilitation. J Hand Surg 2006;31:126–32.

75. Hoang-Kin A, Pegreffi F, Moroni A, et al. Measuring wrist and hand function: common scales and checklists. Injury 2011;42:253–8.

76. Shauver MJ, Chung KC. The minimally clinically important difference of the Michigan Hand Outcome Questionnaire. J Hand Surg Am 2009;34:509–14.

77. Waljee JF, Kim HM, Burns PB, et al. Development of a brief, 12-item version of the Michigan Hand Questionnaire. Plast Reconstr Surg 2011;128:208–20.

78. Levine DW, Simmons BP, Koris MJ, et al. A self-administered questionnaire for the assessment of severity of symptoms and functional status in carpal tunnel syndrome. J Bone Joint Surg Am 1993;75:1585–92.

79. Amadio PC, Silverstein MD, Ilstrup DM, et al. Outcome assessment for carpal tunnel surgery: the relative responsiveness of generic, arthritis-specific, disease-specific and physical examination measures. J Hand Surg Am 1996;21:338–46.

80. Atroshi I, Gummesson C, Johnsson R, et al. Symptoms of disability and quality of life in patients with carpal tunnel syndrome. J Hand Surg Am 1999;24:398–404.

81. Heybeli N, Kutluhan S, Demirci S, et al. Assessment of outcome of carpal tunnel syndrome: a comparison of electrophysiological findings and a self-administered Boston questionnaire. J Hand Surg Am 2002;27:259–64.

82. Mondelli M, Reale F, Sicurelli F, et al. Relationship between the self-administered Boston questionnaire

and electrophysiological findings in follow-up of surgically-treated carpal tunnel syndrome. J Hand Surg Br 2000;25:128–34.

83. Leite JC, Jerosch-Herold C, Song F. A systematic review of the psychometric properties of the Boston Carpal Tunnel Questionnaire. BMC Musculoskelet Disord 2006;7:1–9.

84. Atroshi I, Johnsson R, Nouhan R, et al. Use of outcome instruments to compare workers' compensation and non-workers' compensation carpal tunnel syndrome. J Hand Surg Am 2000; 22:882–8.

85. Ruijs AC, Jaquet JB, Van Riel WG, et al. Cold intolerance following median and ulnar nerve injuries: prognosis and predictors. J Hand Surg Am 2007; 32:434–9.

86. Novak CB, Anastakis DJ, Beaton DE, et al. Cold intolerance after brachial plexus nerve injury. Hand 2012;7:66–71.

87. Stratford P, Gill C, Westaway M, et al. Assessing disability and change on individual patients: a report of a patient specific measure. Physiother Can 1995;47:258–62.

88. Hefford C, Abbot JH, Arnold R, et al. The patient-specific functional scale: validity, reliability, and responsiveness in patients with upper extremity musculoskeletal problems. J Orthop Sports Phys Ther 2012;42:56–65.

89. Novak CB, Anastakis DJ, Beaton DE, et al. Validity of the Patient Specific Functional Scale in patients following upper extremity nerve injury. Hand 2013; 8:132–8.

Tendon Versus Nerve Transfers in Elbow, Wrist, and Hand Reconstruction: A Literature Review

Clifton G. Meals, MD[a],*, Roy A. Meals, MD[b]

KEYWORDS

- Nerve transfer • Tendon transfer • Reconstruction • Upper extremity • Brachial plexus

KEY POINTS

- Brachial plexus injuries are often devastating.
- Reconstruction must be individualized.
- Many procedures for reconstruction exist.
- Robust data facilitating the comparison between individual procedures (particularly tendon and nerve transfer) are sparse.
- Reconstructive decision making is based on surgeon experience and popular consensus rather than excellent evidence.

INTRODUCTION TO BRACHIAL PLEXUS INJURY AND UPPER EXTREMITY RECONSTRUCTION

The hand and arm are uniquely adapted to both sense and manipulate the environment. With brachial plexus injury, higher-order functioning is lost as is the upper extremity's role in nutrition, hygiene, and protection.

Several neurosurgical techniques have been developed for reanimation of the upper extremity: nerve repair, nerve grafting, and nerve transfer. Musculotendinous techniques include free muscle transfer and tendon transfer. These procedures are typically combined and may be accompanied by arthrodesis of the wrist or shoulder to maximize postoperative function.

No two injuries to the brachial plexus are alike. These injuries are typically high-velocity injuries resulting from car or motorcycle accidents, and

injury is expected not only to nerves but also to muscle, vessels, bone, and other organ systems. As with any reconstructive effort, the surgeon must assess the patient's deficits, their remaining function, and the tissue available for reconstruction. An operative strategy is then developed on a case-by-case basis.

The following clinical scenario is used to demonstrate the complexity of such a case:

A 23-year-old man is involved in a high-speed motorcycle collision. On presentation to the emergency department, he has a right-sided hemothorax and multiple broken ribs, an open left tibia fracture, a deep laceration to the right forearm, and no neurologic function in his right upper extremity.

He is intubated; a chest tube is placed; and he is admitted to the intensive care unit. The following morning, his lower extremity injury is

Disclosure: The authors of this article have no conflicts of interest to disclose. This article has not been previously published or submitted in whole or part.
[a] Department of Orthopedics, George Washington University Medical Center, 2170 Pennsylvania Avenue NW, Washington, DC 20037, USA; [b] Department of Orthopedics, University of California Los Angeles Medical Center, 1033 Gayley Avenue #104, Los Angeles, CA 90024, USA
* Corresponding author.
E-mail address: cliftongm@gmail.com

debrided and treated with an intramedullary nail. Exploration of the forearm wound reveals multiple tendon lacerations, which are repaired. Over the following week, the patient's thoracic injury is stabilized, and he is eventually extubated. The right arm is placed in a splint, and the patient is discharged to a rehabilitation facility 3 weeks after his injury.

An outpatient examination 2 weeks later reveals mild atrophy of the right upper extremity. The patient's shoulder is densely numb as is the radial half of the forearm extending to the thumb. He has paresthesias in the index and long finger and intact sensation in the ring and small fingers. The patient elevates his scapula but has no motor function at the shoulder, and he is unable to flex his elbow. He has Medical Research Council (MRC) grade 3 of 5 extension of the elbow, 3 of 5 flexion and extension of the wrist, 3 of 5 flexion and extension of the fingers, and full power of the intrinsic musculature. The patient is interested in surgery to "give him his arm back."

This patient would be a candidate for a combination of carefully chosen procedures; ideally, an evidenced-based approach to treatment would be used. At present, however, the selection of even one particular procedure over another is more a matter of surgeon preference than an evidence-based decision. Belzberg and colleagues[1] have documented the different attitudes toward brachial plexus injuries among experienced surgeons. This lack of consensus is understandable. Given the variety of confounding variables associated with brachial plexus injury, systematic comparison of reconstructive techniques is difficult or impossible. Available data exist largely in the form of retrospective case series (level IV evidence). Only a few retrospective reports directly comparing one technique with another have been published. Merrel and colleagues'[2–4] comparison of different nerve transfers, Garg and colleagues' comparison of nerve transfer and nerve grafts, and Yang and colleagues' comparison of nerve transfer and nerve repair are notable examples.

In the same spirit, the authors performed a review of series describing tendon and nerve transfer for upper extremity reconstruction.

HISTORY OF TENDON AND NERVE TRANSFERS
Tendon Transfer

In the mid nineteenth century, Velpeau and Malgaigne[5,6] both recommended that severed tendons be used to reinforce their intact, adjacent counterparts. In 1881, Nicoladoni[7] recommended the first true transfer of tendon for the purpose of reanimation. Nicoladoni's first attempted tendon transfer (in the foot) failed; however, the idea of transferring tendons gained traction in early twentieth century Europe with the outbreak of polio.[8,9] In 1899, Franke and Capellen both produced early reports of tendon transfer for the restoration of hand function. Sir Robert Jones advocated the transfer of the pronator teres to the extensor carpi radialis longus and brevis in the early twentieth century.[10–12] In 1919, Steindler[13] described a tendon transfer for elbow flexion.[13] Both the Steindler flexorplasty and variants of the Jones transfer are used today. Bunnell[14] developed tendon transfers to treat battlefield injuries after World War I, and much later work in upper extremity reconstruction is based on his experience.[14,15] Today, trauma to nerves and tendons, along with rheumatoid arthritis and other systemic causes of tendon ruptures, are the most common indications for tendon transfer.

Nerve Transfer

Using roosters in the 1820s, Flourens[16] famously demonstrated that nerves in the brachial plexus could be redirected, resulting in the recovery of motor function by nonanatomic neurologic control. Several human experiments followed. At the start of the twentieth century, Balance and colleagues[17] were the first to describe successful motor nerve transfer of the spinal accessory nerve to the facial nerve. Successful nerve transfers both for reanimation and sensation were documented in the mid twentieth century. Brandt and Mackinnon's[18] and Oberlin and colleagues'[19] work renewed enthusiasm for nerve transfers in the 1990s.[18–20] Concurrent technical improvements in electrical diagnosis and microsurgery have made nerve transfer increasingly attractive in cases when macroprocedures might previously have been used.[4,21] With the expansion of this technique has come an expansion of jargon. The terms *nerve transfer*, *nerve suture*, and *nerve crossing* all refer to the heterotopic transfer of a functioning nerve to a nerve that has lost connection to the central nervous system. *Neurotization* is an ambiguous term that best describes the transfer of a nerve directly to muscle.[22]

METHODS

The authors performed a literature review of published case series using the PubMed database. Case series were identified using appropriate key words and then screened based on article title, abstract, or content. Bibliographies of the selected articles as well as those of appropriate review articles were screened to ensure a comprehensive search. Selected series met the following search criteria:

- Reported in English
- Reported primary tendon or nerve transfers for the elbow, wrist, or hand
- Reported procedures indicated for trauma to the peripheral nervous system
- Reported single procedure for each desired movement
- Does not involve the use of interpositional grafts (nerve or tendon)
- Describe 10 or more patients
- Reported cases with surgical delay less than or equal to 1 year (nerve transfers only)
- Reported outcomes about the MRC grading system or facilitating translation to the MRC grading system
- Reported follow-up of 1 year or more
- Not duplicated in other reports

RESULTS

The authors identified 26 case series (in 20 articles) meeting the criteria. Their findings are summarized in **Tables 1** and **2**.

- Elbow flexion
  - Nerve transfers: The authors identified 13 case series meeting the criteria. Eight series described the transfer of intercostal nerves to the musculocutaneous nerve.[23–30] The number of transferred intercostal nerves ranged from 2 to 4 (one article does not explicitly state the number of transferred nerves).[23] Among the 239 patients so treated, 104 (44%) demonstrated elbow flexion greater than or equal to 4 of 5. The portion of patients achieving 3 of 5 power was not universally reported. Five series described the transfer of ulnar nerve fascicles to the musculocutaneous nerve (Oberlin's transfer).[30–34] Among 99 patients treated in this way, 81 (82%) demonstrated elbow flexion greater than or equal to 4 of 5. Thirteen (13%) patients achieved 3 of 5 flexion of the elbow but not greater.
  - Tendon transfers: One series meeting the criteria was identified. Segal and colleagues[35] reported 4 of 5 elbow flexion in 4 of 17 (24%) patients treated with Clark's pectoral muscle transplantation.[36] Seven of 17 (41%) patients achieved elbow flexion of 3 of 5 but not greater.[35]
- Elbow extension
  - Nerve transfers: Two case series meeting the criteria were identified. Each of the 2 series identified describes the transfer of

2 or 3 intercostal nerves to the triceps branch of the radial nerve.[37,38] Among the 25 patients so treated, 9 (36%) achieved elbow extension greater than or equal to 4 of 5. Six of 35 (17%) demonstrated extension strength of 3 of 5 but not greater. Of note, a third relevant series was identified but not included in the authors' evaluation because it seemed to describe patients that were subsequently reported again by the same investigators.[39]
  - Tendon transfers: No series meeting the criteria were identified.
- Wrist flexion
  - Nerve transfers: One case series meeting the criteria was identified. The investigators described the transfer of 2 intercostal nerves to the median nerve in 10 patients. Two of 10 patients achieved wrist flexion of 4 of 5 or greater. Four of 10 patients regained 3 of 5 strength but not greater.[25]
  - Tendon transfers: No series meeting the criteria were identified.
- Wrist Extension
  - Nerve transfers: One case series meeting the criteria was identified. Seventeen patients underwent transfer of fascicles of the median nerve to the radial nerve. Sixteen of 17 patients (94%) regained 4 of 5 strength in wrist extension, and no patients achieved 3 of 5 strength.[40]
  - Tendon transfers: No series meeting the criteria were identified.
- Pronosupination
  - Nerve transfers: No series meeting the criteria were identified.
  - Tendon transfers: No series meeting the criteria were identified.
- Extrinsic finger flexion
  - Nerve transfer: One case series meeting the criteria was identified. Ten patients underwent transfer of 2 intercostal nerves to the median nerve. Two of 10 patients regained 4 of 5 flexion power and 2 of 10 regained 3 of 5 power but not greater.[25]
  - Tendon transfer: One case series meeting the criteria was identified. Thirteen patients underwent transfer of the extensor carpi radialis longus tendon to the flexor digitorum profundus tendon. The investigators reported the return of 4 of 5 finger flexion strength in all patients.[41]
- Finger extension
  - Nerve transfers: Two case series meeting the criteria were identified. Ten patients underwent transfer of the phrenic nerve to the lower trunk of the brachial plexus. Three of

Table 1
Nerve transfers

Source/Motion/Year	Donor Nerve/s	Target Nerve	N	% ≥ M4	M4 > % ≥ M3
Elbow Flexion					
Chuang et al,[24] 1992	ICs (2–3)	MC	66	67	n/a
Ochiai et al,[23] 1993	IC (n/a)	MC	21	24	54
Ogino & Naito,[25] 1995	ICs (2)	MC	10	70	20
Ruch et al,[26] 1995	ICs (2–3)	MC	14	36	0
Malessy & Thomeer,[27] 1998	ICs (2–4)	MC	25	56	8
Okinaga & Nagano,[28] 1999	ICs (2)	MC	11	64	36
Waikakul et al,[29] 1999	ICs (3)	MC	75	20	n/a
Coulet et al,[30] 2010	ICs (3)	MC	17	41	29
Sungpet et al,[34] 2000	U	MC	36	83	11
Bertelli & Ghizoni,[31] 2004	U	MC	10	70	30
Leechavengvongs et al,[32] 2006	U	MC	15	87	13
Venkatramani et al,[33] 2008	U	MC	15	87	13
Coulet et al,[30] 2010	U	MC	23	78	9
Elbow Extension					
Doi et al,[37] 1997	ICs (2)	R	14	14	29
Goubier et al,[38] 2011	ICs (3)	R	11	64	18
Wrist Flexion					
Ogino & Naito,[25] 1995	ICs (2)	M	10	20	40
Wrist Extension					
Ray & Mackinnon,[40] 2011	M	R	17	94	0
Pronosupination					
None					
Extrinsic Finger Flexion					
Ogino & Naito,[25] 1995	ICs (2)	M	10	20	20
Finger Extension					
Lin et al,[42] 2011	Ph	BP (LT)	10	30	50
Ray & Mackinnon,[40] 2011	M	R	19	58	11
Thumb Extension					
Lin et al,[42] 2011	Ph	BP (LT)	10	10	60
Ray & Mackinnon,[40] 2011	M	R	19	58	11
Thumb Pinch					
n/a					
Hand Intrinsics					
n/a					

Abbreviations: BP, brachial plexus; ICs (n), intercostal nerves (number transferred); LT, lower trunk; M, median nerve; MC, musculocutaneous nerve; Ph, phrenic nerve; R, radial nerve; U, ulnar nerve.

10 patients achieved 4 of 5 motor power, and 5 of 10 patients regained 3 of 5 power but not greater.[42] A second series described transfer of fascicles of the median nerve to the radial nerve. Eleven of 19 patients (58%) regained 4 of 5 motor power, and 2 of 19 patients (11%) achieved 3 of 5 strength but not greater.[40]

○ Tendon transfers: One case series meeting the criteria was identified. Twenty-nine patients underwent transfer of flexor digitorum superficialis slips to the extensor digitorum communis, extensor indicis proprius (EIP), and extensor pollicis longus (EPL). All 29 patients so treated regained 3 of 5 extension strength.[43]

Table 2
Tendon transfers

Source/Motion/Year	Donor Tendon	Target Tendon	N	% ≥ M4	M4 > % ≥ M3
Elbow Flexion					
Segal et al,[35] 1959	Pectoralis major	Biceps	17	24	41
Elbow Extension					
n/a					
Wrist Flexion					
n/a					
Wrist Extension					
n/a					
Pronosupination					
n/a					
Extrinsic Finger Flexion					
Goubier & Teboul,[41] 2008	ECRL	FDP	13	100	0
Finger Extension					
Krishnan & Schackert,[43] 2008	FDS (long, ring)	EIP, EPL, EDC	29	n/a	100
Thumb Extensors					
n/a					
Thumb Opposition					
Anderson et al,[46] 1991	EIP	APB, EPL	16	n/a	100
Thumb Pinch					
n/a					

Abbreviations: APB, abductor pollicis brevis; ECRL, extensor carpi radialis longus; EDC, extensor digitorum communis; EIP, extensor indicis proprius; EPL, extensor pollicis longus; FDP, flexor digitorum profundus; FDS, flexor digitorum superficialis; n/a, not available.

- Thumb extension
  - Nerve transfers: Two case series meeting the criteria were identified. Ten patients underwent transfer of the phrenic nerve to the lower trunk of the brachial plexus. One of 10 patients regained 4 of 5 strength, and 7 of 10 patients achieved 3 of 5 motor power but not greater.[42] A second series described transfer of fascicles of the median nerve to the radial nerve. Of the patients so treated, 11 of 19 (58%) regained 4 of 5 motor power and 2 of 19 (11%) regained 3 of 5 strength but not greater.[40]
  - Tendon transfers: No series meeting the criteria were identified.
- Thumb opposition
  - Nerve transfers: No series meeting the criteria were identified.
  - Tendon transfers: One case series meeting the criteria was identified. The investigators described transfer of the EIP to the abductor pollicis brevis, the EPL, and the metacarpophalangeal joint capsule in 16 patients, all of whom regained 3 of 5 strength.

- Thumb pinch
  - Nerve transfers: No series meeting the criteria were identified.
  - Tendon transfers: No series meeting the criteria were identified.
- Intrinsic function (metacarpophalangeal joint flexion, interphalangeal joint extension, finger abduction and adduction)
  - Nerve transfers: No series meeting the criteria were identified.
  - Tendon transfers: No series meeting the criteria were identified.

DISCUSSION

Compared with that of similar reports,[2–4] the authors' search criterion was relatively strict. Reports of nerve or tendon transfers as secondary or salvage procedures were eschewed to minimize confounding. For the same reason, the authors excluded series reporting the use of interpositional nerve or tendon grafts as well as reports of simultaneous procedures for reanimation of a single motion (e.g., concurrent Steindler flexorplasty and

Oberlin nerve transfer for elbow flexion). (Cases describing arthrodesis of an adjacent joint were permitted.) Likewise, nontraumatic indications for surgery (eg, tetraplegia, stroke, cerebral and obstetric palsy, polio, rheumatoid arthritis, and leprosy) were avoided as were cases of nerve transfer surgery more than 1 year after injury. To maximize the reliability of the selected data, the authors rejected series with fewer than 10 patients and less than 1 year of follow-up. Selected studies all used either the MRC grading scale or reported data so that results could be interpreted in terms of the MRC scale; this facilitated a fair comparison.

The selected articles represent only a small fraction of available, relevant literature on the subject. Nonetheless, the authors' goal was a comparison between objective, reliable outcome data collected after tendon or nerve transfer. Ultimately, the authors are forced to present their conclusion as a pertinent negative: objective comparison between tendon and nerve transfers for upper extremity reconstruction is difficult or impossible given then paucity of reliable data on the subject.

The most robust data the authors did uncover pertained to nerve transfers for elbow flexion. This finding reflects the thought that elbow flexion should take priority in upper extremity reconstruction, followed by shoulder abduction and external rotation, scapular stabilization, elbow extension, and then function of the wrist and hand.[44] The authors' amalgamated data on transfer of intercostal nerves to the musculocutaneous nerve suggests that less than half of patients so treated regain useful flexion of the elbow. Grouped data pertaining to the transfer of ulnar nerve fascicles to the musculocutaneous nerve (Oberlin transfer) suggest that this transfer is somewhat more reliable.

The Steindler flexorplasty (proximal advancement of the flexor-pronator origin) may be the most popular tendon-based procedure for restoration of elbow flexion. Although the authors accepted several articles describing nerve transfers for elbow flexion, they found no articles describing the Steindler operation that met their search criteria. The authors speculate that this disparity exists because nerve transfers have emerged in an era of more rigorous publication standards. The Steindler operation persists, nonetheless, on the strength of experience and popular consensus.

Although the Steindler operation and its counterparts remain popular, there are several appealing aspects of nerve transfer: (1) Nerve transfers may better preserve anatomy. Nerve transfers may preserve physiologic muscle balance at the wrist, for instance, as opposed to flexor-to-extensor tendon transfers that necessarily disrupt this relationship. More rapid neurologic relearning may be a related benefit.[44] (2) Nerve transfers may involve less donor site morbidity. (3) Nerve transfers may be undertaken outside of the zone of injury.[44,45] (4) Nerve transfers may be used to restore protective sensation and to relieve neuropathic pain.[44]

A distinct *dis*advantage of nerve transfer is that it is unlikely to succeed beyond 12 to 18 months after the injury when target motor end plates have degenerated.[45]

Given these considerations, we can return to the case example and suggest a course of treatment. Given the damage to the patient's forearm musculature and his 3 of 5 flexion power at the wrist, the flexor-pronator mass is an unattractive donor, and an Oberlin transfer seems relatively advantageous. Intact lower roots of the brachial plexus and clinical preservation of the intrinsic muscles make the ulnar nerve a viable donor. This procedure avoids a more proximal transfer, extended dissection, and prolonged reinnervation time. Direct distal transfer also obviates nerve grafting, again shortening the predicted time to recovery. Although the authors are unable to objectively compare tendon and nerve transfer for elbow flexion based on their review, they did uncover solid evidence in support of the Oberlin transfer. The authors echo the attitude of Lee and Wolfe[44] who suggest that tendon transfer be used in this scenario only after the nerve transfer has failed.

The authors' strict selection criteria reveal the true scarcity of high-level evidence on the subject. There are several weaknesses of this review. (1) In many cases, especially in regard to distal tendon transfers, the authors were forced to translate outcome measures, typically range of motion, into an MRC score. It would be unfair to assume that active range of motion represented 4 of 5 strength, rather the authors translated this finding into 3 of 5 power and may have considerably underestimated the success of these procedures. (2) Because many of the articles the authors reviewed did not report preoperative strength, they account only for absolute rather than relative recovery of joint function. (3) In an effort to isolate individual reconstructive techniques, the authors excluded series describing multiple simultaneous procedures for restoration of a single function (eg, transfer of ulnar and median nerve fascicles to the biceps and brachialis motor branches). These dual procedures are not uncommon and are, in fact, preferred by some investigators.[44] (4) The authors' review casts little light on other common scenarios in upper extremity reconstruction: central nervous system trauma, obstetric palsy, cerebral palsy, polio, and so forth.

SUMMARY

Upper extremity surgeons have several reconstructive procedures at their disposal, among them tendon and nerve transfers. A truly objective comparison of these procedures at the elbow, wrist, and hand is impossible given the scarcity of robust data on the subject. Tendon transfers have a long history; their continued use is founded in surgeon familiarity, anecdotal reports, and experience. Although nerve transfers have emerged in an era of improved reporting, time has not permitted the collection of excellent data on the subject. As such, a major aspect of reconstructive decision making remains more a matter of art than science.

REFERENCES

1. Belzberg A, Dorsi M, Storm P, et al. Surgical repair of brachial plexus injury: a multinational survey of experienced peripheral nerve surgeons. J Neurosurg 2004;101:365–76.
2. Garg R, Merrell G, Hillstrom H, et al. Comparison of nerve transfers and nerve grafting for traumatic upper plexus palsy: a systematic review and analysis. J Bone Joint Surg Am 2011;93:819–29.
3. Yang L, Chang K, Chung K. A systematic review of nerve transfer and nerve repair for the treatment of adult upper brachial plexus injury. Neurosurgery 2012;71:417–29.
4. Merrell G, Barrie K, Katz D, et al. Results of nerve transfer techniques for restoration of shoulder and elbow function in the context of a meta-analysis of the English literature. J Hand Surg Am 2001;26:303–14.
5. Velpeau A. Elements de medecine operatoire. Augmente d'un traite des bandages de petite chirurgie. Paris: JB Bailliere; 1839.
6. Malgaigne J. Memoire sur la valeur reele de l'orthopedie et specialment de la myotomie rachidienne dans le traitement de deviations laterales de l'epine. Paris: JB Bailliere; 1845.
7. Nicoladoni CÜ. Sehnentransplantation. Aus der chirurgischen Section 54. Versammlung deutscher Naturforscher und Aerzte in Salzburg. Arch Gynecol Obstet. 1881;18:463–97.
8. Sammer D, Chung K. Tendon transfers: part 1. Principles of transfer and transfers for radial nerve palsy. Plast Reconstr Surg 2009;123:169e–77e.
9. Agostini T, Lazzeri D. Tendon transfer in radial palsy: a historical reappraisal. Plast Reconstr Surg 2010; 126:1796–7.
10. Raskin K, Wilgis E. Flexor carpi ulnaris transfer for radial nerve palsy: functional testing of long-term results. J Hand Surg Am 1995;20:737–42.
11. Jones R. On suture of nerves, and alternative methods of treatment by transplantation of tendon. BMJ 1916;1:641–3.
12. Jones R. Tendon transplantation in cases of musculospiral injuries not amenable to suture. Am J Surg 1921;35:333–5.
13. Steindler A. Operative treatment of paralytic conditions of the upper extremity. J Bone Joint Surg Am 1919;1:608–19.
14. Bunnell S. Reconstructive surgery of the hand. Surg Gynecol Obstet 1924;39:259–74.
15. Wolfe S, editor. Green's operative hand surgery. 6 edition. Philadephia: Elsevier; 2010.
16. Flourens M. Experiences sur la reunion ou cicatrisation des plaies de la Moelle epiniere et des Nerfs. Ann Science Nat 1828;13:113–22.
17. Ballance C, Ballance H, Stewart P. Remarks on the operative treatment of chronic facial palsy of peripheral origin. Br Med J 1903;1:1009–13.
18. Brandt K, Mackinnon S. A technique for maximizing biceps recovery in brachial plexus reconstruction. J Hand Surg 1993;18:726–33.
19. Oberlin C, Béal D, Leechavengvongs S, et al. Nerve transfer to biceps muscle using a part of ulnar nerve for C5-C6 avulsion of the brachial plexus: anatomical study and report of four cases. J Hand Surg Am 1994;19:232–7.
20. Wong A, Pianta T, Mastella D. Nerve transfers. Hand Clin 2012;28:571–7.
21. Spinner R, Shin A, Hebert-Blouin M, et al. Traumatic brachial plexus injury. In: Wolfe S, editor. Green's operative hand surgery. Philadelphia: Churhill Livingstone: Elsevier; 2010. p. 1235–92.
22. Meals R, Nelissen R. The origin and meaning of "neurotization". J Hand Surg Am 1995;20:144–6.
23. Ochiai N, Mikami Y, Yamamoto S, et al. A new technique for mismatched nerve suture in direct intercostal nerve transfers. J Hand Surg Br 1993;18:318–9.
24. Chuang D, Yeh M, Wei F. Intercostal nerve transfer of the musculocutaneous nerve in avulsed brachial plexus injuries: evaluation of 66 patients. J Hand Surg Am 1992;17:822–8.
25. Ogino T, Naito T. Intercostal nerve crossing to restore elbow flexion and sensibility of the hand for a root avulsion type of brachial plexus injury. Microsurgery 1995;16:571–7.
26. Ruch D, Friedman A, Nunley J. The restoration of elbow flexion with intercostal nerve transfers. Clin Orthop 1995;314:95–103.
27. Malessy M, Thomeer R. Evaluation of intercostal to musculocutaneous nerve transfer in reconstructive brachial plexus surgery. J Neurosurg 1998;88:266–71.
28. Okinaga S, Nagano A. Can vascularization improve the surgical outcome of the intercostal nerve transfer for traumatic brachial plexus palsy? A clinical comparison of vascularized and non-vascularized methods. Microsurgery 1999;19:176–80.
29. Waikakul S, Wongtragul S, Vanadurongwan V. Restoration of elbow flexion in brachial plexus

avulsion injury: comparing spinal accessory nerve transfer with intercostal nerve transfer. J Hand Surg Am 1999;24:571–7.

30. Coulet B, Boretto J, Lazerges C, et al. A comparison of intercostal and partial ulnar nerve transfers in restoring elbow flexion following upper brachial plexus injury (C5-C6+/-C7). J Hand Surg Am 2010;35:1297–303.

31. Bertelli J, Ghizoni M. Reconstruction of C5 and C6 brachial plexus avulsion injury by multiple nerve transfers: spinal accessory to suprascapular, ulnar fascicles to biceps branch, and triceps long or lateral head branch to axillary nerve. J Hand Surg Am 2004;29:131–9.

32. Leechavengvongs S, Witoonchart K, Uerpairojkit C, et al. Combined nerve transfers for C5 and C6 brachial plexus avulsion injury. J Hand Surg Am 2006;31:183–9.

33. Venkatramani H, Bhardwaj P, Faruquee S, et al. Functional outcome of nerve transfer for restoration of shoulder and elbow function in upper brachial plexus injury. J Brachial PLex Peripher Nerve Inj 2008;3:15.

34. Sungpet A, Suphachatwong C, Kawinwonggowit V, et al. Transfer of a single fascicle from the ulnar nerve to the biceps muscle after avulsions of upper roots of the brachial plexus. J Hand Surg Br 2000; 25:325–8.

35. Segal A, Seddon H, Brooks D. Treatment of paralysis of the flexors of the elbow. J Bone Joint Surg Br 1959;41:44–50.

36. Clark J. Reconstruction of biceps brachii by pectoral muscle transplantation. Br J Surg 1946;34:180.

37. Doi K, Shigetomi M, Kaneko K, et al. Significance of elbow extension in reconstruction of prehension with reinnervated free-muscle transfer following complete brachial plexus avulsion. Plast Reconstr Surg 1997;100:364–72.

38. Goubier J, Teboul F, Khalifa H. Reanimation of elbow extension with intercostal nerves transfers in total brachial plexus palsies. Microsurgery 2011; 31:7–11.

39. Goubier J, Teboul F. Transfer of the intercostal nerves to the nerve of the long head of the triceps to recover elbow extension in brachial plexus palsy. Tech Hand Up Extrem Surg 2007;11:139–41.

40. Ray W, Mackinnon S. Clinical outcomes following median to radial nerve transfers. J Hand Surg Am 2011;36:201–8.

41. Goubier J, Teboul F. Management of hand palsies in isolated C7 to T1 or C8, T1 root avulsions. Tech Hand Up Extrem Surg 2008;12:156–60.

42. Lin H, Hou C, Chen A, et al. Transfer of the phrenic nerve to the posterior division of the lower trunk to recover thumb and finger extension in brachial plexus palsy. J Neurosurg 2011;114:212–6.

43. Krishnan K, Schackert G. An analysis of results after selective tendon transfers through the interosseous membrane to provide selective finger and thumb extension in chronic irreparable radial nerve lesions. J Hand Surg Am 2008;33:223–31.

44. Lee S, Wolfe S. Nerve transfers for the upper extremity: new horizons in nerve reconstruction. J Am Acad Orthop Surg 2012;20:506–17.

45. Tung T, Mackinnon S. Nerve transfers: indications, techniques, and outcomes. J Hand Surg Am 2010; 35:332–41.

46. Anderson G, Lee V, Sundararaj G. Extensor indicis proprius opponensplasty. J Hand Surg Br 1991;16: 334–8.

Management of Chronic Pain Following Nerve Injuries/CRPS Type II

Ian Carroll, MD, MS[a], Catherine M. Curtin, MD[b,c],*

KEYWORDS

- Chronic pain • Complex regional pain syndrome • Neuropathic pain • Nerve injuries

KEY POINTS

- Perioperative interventions can reduce incidence of postoperative chronic pain: prevention is much more desirable than treating complex regional pain syndrome (CRPS)/neuropathic pain.
- There is a critical time window in treating the patient with CRPS/neuropathic pain: early intervention is better.
- Surgeons need to be comfortable beginning treatment of CRPS/neuropathic pain.

Every incision and every fracture injures some sensory nerve. Most of the time, these nerves recover from this insult without long-term consequences; however, for some people, pain continues long after the wounds have healed. This chronic pain then affects quality of life, limits the patient's ability to participate in therapy, and adversely affects functional outcomes. Chronic postoperative pain is a particularly frustrating problem for the surgeon because it is hard to anticipate, ruins a technically perfect procedure, and the surgeon may be unsure of the next steps of treatment. There is much information on chronic pain and its treatment, but this literature is often published outside of surgery and diffusion of this information across disciplines is slow. This article synthesizes some of this literature and provides a systematic presentation of the evidence on pain associated with peripheral nerve injury.

Chronic pain and complex regional pain syndrome (CRPS) are large topics and we have divided this article into sections. When available, we have presented pooled data for each subsection, including consensus statements and systematic reviews. When pooled data are not available,

we present information from randomized controlled trials (RCTs). Given the diversity and the breadth of the topic, we hope that this overview provides an information foundation and the reviews presented will direct the reader to more detailed information.

DEFINITIONS

The first step when discussing pain is to understand terminology.

Neuropathic Pain

This article focuses on pain associated with nerve injuries: neuropathic pain. The International Association for the Study of Pain (IASP) Neuropathic Pain Special Interest Group has defined neuropathic pain arising as a direct consequence of a lesion or disease affecting the somatosensory system.[1,2] It has typical characteristics that help separate it from other types of pain, such as joint pain from osteoarthritis. A recent Delphi survey of experts defined neuropathic pain as having a clinical history of nerve injury and the pain should demonstrate typical characteristics: (1) prickling, tingling, pins

a Department of Anesthesia, Stanford University, 450 Broadway, Redwood City, CA 94603, USA; b Department of Surgery, Palo Alto VA, 3801 Miranda Avenue, Palo Alto VA, Palo Alto, CA 94304, USA; c Division of Plastic Surgery, Stanford University, Suite 400, 770 Welch RD Palo Alto, CA 94304, USA
* Corresponding author. Division of Plastic Surgery, Stanford University, Suite 400, 770 Welch RD Palo Alto, CA 94304.
E-mail address: curtincatherine@yahoo.com

Hand Clin 29 (2013) 401–408
http://dx.doi.org/10.1016/j.hcl.2013.04.009
0749-0712/13/$ – see front matter © 2013 Elsevier Inc. All rights reserved.

hand.theclinics.com

and needles; (2) pain with light touch; (3) electric shocks or shooting pain; (4) hot or burning pain; and (5) Brush allodynia.[3] For the researcher, there are several validated measures to differentiate neuropathic pain.[4] For more detailed information on how to assess neuropathic pain, we refer you to a recent guideline, which provides detailed information on recommended measures.[5]

Chronic Pain

Acute pain after injury is a normal and healthy response. It serves the purpose of limiting activity and protecting the injured areas to allow the tissue to heal. Yet at some point, pain transitions to a pathologic process, no longer serving the protective role, and the pain becomes chronic or intractable. Much effort has been devoted to define when pain has transitioned to this chronic state. Smith and colleagues'[3] consensus study felt neuropathic pain was intractable when the pain persisted despite trials of at least 4 drugs of known effectiveness in neuropathic pain. The most frequently cited definition for chronic pain was produced by the IASP, which states that chronic pain is pain that has persisted beyond the normal tissue healing time and often 3 months is set as the convenient cutoff.[1]

CRPS

The definition of complex regional pain has undergone a long evolution as our understanding of the process has evolved. During the Civil War era, it was known as causalgia. In 1946, this type of pain was referred to as Reflex Sympathetic Dystrophy,[6] and during the 1990s, the nomenclature was changed to the current term: CRPS. There has been much debate on the criteria to make this diagnosis. Both the IASP and a consensus statement called the Budapest criteria present fairly similar lists of what a patient should display to have a diagnosis of CRPS.[7,8] The IASP defines CRPS as a syndrome characterized by a continuing (spontaneous and/or evoked) regional pain that is seemingly disproportionate in time or degree to the usual course of pain after trauma or other lesion. The pain is regional (not in a specific nerve territory or dermatome) and usually has a distal predominance of abnormal sensory, motor, sudomotor, vasomotor edema, and/or trophic findings.[7] This article focuses on the CRPS type II associated with nerve injury; however, it is not hard to imagine that CRPS type I may be mediated by similar pathways by injury to smaller unnamed nerves in the bone and soft tissue.

This diagnosis of CRPS is based on history and physical examination: there is no specific diagnostic test for CRPS. Given that CRPS is a clinical diagnosis, there has been a much research on what clinical signs are most specific to this diagnosis. The IASP guidelines state that the patient must have pain disproportionate to the injury and there is no other diagnosis that explains the pain. **Box 1** presents the most recent clinical criteria for diagnosis of CRPS.[8]

EPIDEMIOLOGY

Severe complex regional pain syndrome is a rare occurrence, but chronic pain after injury to sensory nerves is more frequent. CRPS may be the severe

---

Box 1
Clinical criteria for complex regional pain syndrome

Must report at least one symptom in 3 of the 4 following categories

1. Sensory: Reports of hyperalgesia and/or allodynia

2. Vasomotor: Reports of temperature asymmetry and/or skin color changes and/or skin color asymmetry

3. Sudomotor/Edema: Reports of edema and/or sweating changes and/or sweating asymmetry

4. Motor/Trophic: Reports of decreased range of motion and/or motor dysfunction (weakness, tremor, dystonia) and/or trophic changes (hair, nail, skin)

Must display at least 1 sign[a] at time of evaluation in at least 2 of the following categories

1. Sensory: Evidence of hyperalgesia (to pinprick) and/or allodynia (to light touch and/or deep somatic pressure and/or joint movement)

2. Vasomotor: Evidence of temperature asymmetry and/or skin color changes and/or asymmetry

3. Sudomotor/Edema: Evidence of edema and/or sweating changes and/or sweating asymmetry

4. Motor/Trophic: Evidence of decreased range of motion and/or motor dysfunction (weakness, tremor, dystonia) and/or trophic changes (hair, nail, skin)

[a] A sign is counted only if it is observed at time of diagnosis.

Data from Harden RN, Oaklander AL, Burton AW, et al. Complex regional pain syndrome: practical diagnostic and treatment guidelines. Pain Med 2013 Feb;14(2):180–229.

end stage of a spectrum of pain processes after nerve injury. Epidemiologic studies of complex regional pain syndrome are often flawed because of the infrequency of the diagnosis. The largest study was from the Netherlands using a general population database.[9] The investigators looked at 217,000 patients and found the overall incidence of CRPS was 26 per 100,000 person years. Women were affected at least 3 times more often than men and the upper extremity was affected more frequently than the lower limb.

Chronic pain after nerve injury is far more common than CRPS. There are no large studies assessing the incidence of pain after major nerve injury. Case series in brachial plexus injuries have found that nearly all patients experience pain after injury. A recent case series of patients with nerve injuries found a high prevalence of pain (66%), with many having severe pain.[10] Yet even smaller injuries, such as the trauma associated with carpal tunnel syndrome, have a 20% rate of pain at 3 months.[11] Although the pain after carpal tunnel release is not a direct nerve injury, the pain is often burning and the scar is sensitive to light touch: features consistent with a neuropathic process. Many of these may be because of injury to branches of the palmar cutaneous branch of the median nerve. Thus, for the hand surgeon, understanding methods to prevent and treat chronic pain associated with a nerve injury is important to improve outcomes.

PREVENTION

The hand surgeon should understand preventive measures that can influence the postoperative pain course and identify the patients/procedures that would be at higher risk for postoperative pain so perioperative measures can be instituted. So who is at risk? There has been extensive work to stratify characteristics associated with the development of chronic pain. First is the type of injury. Major nerve trauma bombards the spinal cord and central nervous system with nociceptive stimuli and, not unexpectedly, these patients are at high risk of pain. Then there are also specific injuries, such as distal radius fracture, which have a high rate of development of CRPS.[12] Patient factors also are associated with risk of chronic pain. CRPS is more frequently seen in women.[9] Psychological factors before injury have long been thought to increase the risk chronic pain. The theory is that a patient with an increased basal rate of catecholamines will be more easily sensitized to pain, but the data are lacking and, at this time, the link between psychological traits and CRPS risk is still speculative.

One of the most important predictors of high postoperative pain is high preoperative pain level: these patients already have a nociceptive system that is primed. Thus, if the surgeon is caring for a patient with several risk factors, it is helpful to consider perioperative interventions.

The next section reviews perioperative interventions that have data from RCTs that support their role in reducing postoperative chronic pain.

Preemptive use of local anesthetics can reduce the number of patients who have chronic postoperative pain. A study on patients who had breast surgery found that the group that received regional anesthetic block had significantly decreased pain at 1 month, 6 months, and 12 months after surgery when compared with the control group.[13] Another trial found decreased pain months after surgery in the group that had a preoperative block before thoracotomy.[14] There are several other studies indicating that anesthetizing the nerve with local analgesia before incision affects long-term chronic pain.[15]

Vitamin C has also been found to reduce the transition to CRPS after distal radius fractures. Vitamin C is a free radical scavenger, which reduces vascular permeability after trauma. It has also may decrease tumor necrosis factor alpha and interleukin-6, which are important inflammatory cytokines. Zollinger and colleagues[16] evaluated vitamin C in the treatment of distal radius fractures in an RCT of 123 patients. They determined 500 mg of vitamin C for 50 days provided a statistical benefit, with decreased pain in these patients. They next looked at dosing study and found that the odds ratio of developing CRPS after distal radius fracture was 0.22 among those who received vitamin C. Statistically significant benefit was seen at 500 mg per day and 1500 mg per day.[17] Another quasiexperimental study on foot and ankle patients found that after institution of a perioperative vitamin C regimen, the rate for CRPS decreased from 9.6% to 1.7%.[18] These 3 studies support the use of vitamin C at 500 mg per day as part of the perioperative regimen.

There are several other medications that show promise for reducing the transition to chronic pain, including gabapentin and ketamine. There are good data for improvement with these medications in acute pain after surgery, but because of wide heterogeneity in the literature, there is still a lack of evidence on their impact on chronic pain. There is a new meta-analysis of gabapentin and pregabalin, supporting their use for chronic pain.[19] At this time, we would advise the surgeon that these medications may reduce chronic pain and the surgeon should consider using these medications despite weaker levels of evidence. Our algorithm for the perioperative management of pain, based on the available literature, is provided in **Tables 1** and **2**.

TREATMENT

Despite the most meticulous care, the surgeon will still be faced with the patient who has lingering chronic pain well after the soft tissue has healed. If the physician feels the patient meets the criteria for CRPS treatment, referral to a pain specialist should be initiated immediately. However, the reality of practice is such that there is often a delay before a pain specialist sees the patient and thus the hand surgeon should start treatment. In addition, the surgeon may have patients with neuropathic pain who do not fully meet the criteria for CRPS but require additional treatment for their pain. The animal studies are clear that there is a window of opportunity with pain; thus, if a patient is having pain disproportionate to expectations, therapy should be initiated promptly in attempt to break the process.[19] The next paragraph reviews evidence-based treatments for chronic neuropathic pain/CRPS.

The surgeon should always begin with a thorough physical examination to rule out treatable causes of the pain, such as carpal tunnel syndrome. There have been several case series that have shown patients who present with CRPS may have a nerve entrapment that responded to surgical release.[20,21] Practitioners should have a low threshold for obtaining additional electrodiagnostic testing if there is a suspicion of nerve entrapments.

Therapy

The first arm of treatment is therapy and other non-pharmacological modalities, which are keystones in neuropathic pain management. The goal is to provide sensory reorganization and desensitization, and extinguish the pathologic pain pathways. There are a few randomized trials demonstrating benefits for therapy when compared with controls.[22–24] Two meta-analyses looking at physical therapy modalities for the treatment of CRPS have been performed. Although these studies were hindered by the heterogeneity of the literature, they did find evidence that graded motor imagery and mirror therapy reduced pain.[25,26] Acupuncture has been studied as an adjunct treatment for chronic pain. At this point, evidence is lacking for the treatment of CRPS but a large study in Germany found that acupuncture reduced pain for a variety of conditions.[27] There are many other modalities that have been described for the treatment of CRPS, but at this time, strong evidence does not exist (eg, myofascial releases, stress loading).

Medications

Pharmacologic treatments are a second arm in management of CRPS and neuropathic pain. During the acute phase of CRPS, corticosteroids have been used as burst therapy, which has been supported in some randomized trials.[28,29] Most other medications that have been studied were in those with a chronic presentation of CRPS/neuropathic pain. A mainstay in treatment for chronic pain is gabapentin, which was originally produced as an antiseizure medication and has become a useful pain management tool.[30] It binds to the alpha-2 delta subunit of presynaptic P/Q-type voltage-gated calcium channels, modulating the traffic and function of these channels. This may directly modulate release of excitatory neurotransmitters from activated nociceptors. Alternatively, some data suggest that gabapentin's antinociceptive mechanism may arise through activation of

Table 1 Authors' perioperative treatment algorithm	
All Patients	1. Preoperative local anesthetic administration (at site of incision or using a block)
Moderate concern for chronic postoperative pain	1. Preoperative local anesthetics 2. Vitamin C 500 mg daily for 50 d
High concern for chronic postoperative pain (patient with high preoperative pain, nerve manipulation, high anxiety)	1. Preoperative local anesthetics 2. Gabapentin 900 mg 2 h before surgery 3. Gabapentin 300–600 mg 3 times a day for 14–30 d (if tolerated by patient) 4. Vitamin C 500 mg daily for 50 d 5. If a general anesthetic: we ask the anesthesiologist about possibility of intraoperative ketamine administration

Table 2
Authors' treatment algorithm for patient presenting with CRPS/neuropathic pain

New acute CRPS	1. Urgent referral to pain specialist
	2. Solumedrol dose pack if acute presentation
	3. Gabapentin 300–1200 mg 3 times a day (as tolerated by patient)[a]
	4. Vitamin C 500 mg/d
	5. Search for occult nerve injury: comprehensive nerve conduction studies and evaluate for sensory nerve injuries easily missed on nerve conduction studies: (1) radial sensory branch injury, (2) palmar cutaneous branch of the median, (3) cutaneous neuromas in scar.
Diffuse neuropathic pain	1. Gabapentin 300–1200 mg 3 times a day (as tolerated by patient)[a]
	2. Desipramine 25 mg and increase each week by 25 mg until taking 100–150 mg/d. Goal is serum plasma level 100–300 ng/mL. Desipramine can have cardiac toxicity at higher doses, thus it is not for patients with heart disease or family history of sudden death, and not for patients taking other antidepressants.
	3. If not candidate for tricyclic antidepressants because of heart disease, consider duloxetine. Start 20 mg/d and increase to 60–120 mg/d.
	4. Start therapy including myofascial releases
Diffuse neuropathic pain (not tolerating or no effect of gabapentin)	1. Desipramine 25 mg and increase each week by 25 mg until taking 100–150 mg/d. Goal is serum plasma level 100–300 ng/mL. Desipramine can have cardiac toxicity at higher doses, thus it is not for patients with heart disease or family history of sudden death, and not for patients taking other antidepressants.
	2. If not candidate for tricyclic antidepressants because of heart disease, consider duloxetine. Start 20 mg/d and increase to 60–120 mg/d.
Tender scar to light touch	1. Inject intradermally with bupivacaine, if relief = scar problem
	2. Therapy for scar management and desensitization
	3. Trial of topicals, such as capsaicin
	4. Potential Botox injection[b]
	5. Consider scar revision if conservative treatment fails
	6. Some scar neuromas are not particularly tender but pain relief occurs with intradermal injection.

[a] Dosing of gabapentin is challenging; there is the balance of getting an efficacious does without having side effects, such as drowsiness, which make the medication intolerable. We titrate up slowly starting 300 mg per day and increasing every other day to a goal of 600 mg 3 times a day. Patients are counseled to stop increasing the dose when side effects become too bothersome (ie, stop at dose they can live with). Some patients just do not tolerate higher doses of gabapentin, we have found that for these patients starting very low (100 mg per day) and slowly titrating up can allow patients to get benefit from this medication.
[b] Botox in painful scars is an off-label use of this medication with only preliminary data at this time.

noradrenergic pain-inhibiting pathways in the spinal cord and brain.[31] Although there are limited data on gabapentin for CRPS, there is a wealth of literature on the treatment of chronic neuropathic pain. A recent Cochrane review looked at gabapentin for those with chronic neuropathic pain and found that gabapentin gave a high level of relief to about a third of the patients with mostly tolerable adverse effects[32]; however one RCT of gabapentin in patients with CRPS I found only mild effect.[33] Gabapentin is a fairly safe medication but has frequent side effects that can be intolerable to the patient. The common side effects are fatigue, dizziness, weight gain, and restlessness. More severe side effects are rare but include changes in mood and suicidal thoughts. We have found that slow initiation of dosing and allowing the patient to hold at the dose where side effects become bothersome has increased patient acceptance of this drug. Pregabalin shares the same mechanism of action and side effects as gabapentin; however, it is absorbed more efficiently by the small intestines when given at higher doses. Switching from gabapentin to pregabalin may therefore be useful in patients who describe partial analgesia at 1200 mg of gabapentin 3 times a day without the occurrence of dose-limiting side effects.

Bisphophonates have some of the best evidence showing benefit in the treatment of CRPS. They were proposed as a treatment for CRPS because they inhibit bone resorption, which is a common finding in patients with CRPS. Several studies have shown benefit from bisphosphonates for CRPS.[34–36] Indeed, a recent review of clinical trials to treat CRPS found that bisphosphonates were the only medications with clear benefits for patients with CRPS.[37] There has been concern that long-term use of bisphosphonates may result in pathologic fractures, but this complication is rare, and for the treatment of CRPS, many patients need only a few months of treatment. Bisphosphonates should be avoided in patients with poor dentition because of the risk of osteonecrosis of the jaw, and patients should be warned to report any jaw, face, tooth, or head discomfort during treatment.

Tricyclic antidepressants (TCAs; amitriptyline, desipramine, and imipramine) are also routinely used in the treatment of neuropathic pain. These medications augment the pain inhibitory pathways and can have other beneficial side effects, such as amitriptyline helping with sleep and desipramine helping with mood. The 2007 Cochrane review confirmed that TCAs were beneficial and these are tolerated well by most patients.[38] Amitriptyline is safe at low doses and can be started while waiting for the patient to be seen by a pain specialist. No one tricyclic is more effective than another, but they all seem to be more effective the higher the dose that the patient is able to tolerate. In this regard, desipramine is particularly helpful because it has the least affinity for the muscarinic cholinergic and histamine receptors that mediate side effects. Patients are therefore often able to tolerate a titration to 100 to 150 mg per day where TCAs are more effective. A typical regimen starts at 25 mg per day and increases by 25 mg each week. However, with high doses there are cardiac side effects. So for the hand surgeon, starting out with 25 mg daily while waiting for a pain specialist is a safe and effective starting strategy.

Topical medications have also been used for chronic pain treatment, including EMLA cream, capsaicin ointment, and lidocaine patches. Capsaicin has good evidence of efficacy in treatment of neuropathic pain. Its mechanism of action was once thought related to substance P but is now thought to arise via the TRPV1 receptor. Overactivation of nociceptors by capsaicin may cause some of these fibers to actually die back from the skin surface. A 1997 meta-analysis of 5 trials determined that capsaicin had a positive effect compared with placebo and a more recent Cochrane review confirmed that capsaicin provided pain relief.[39,40]

Interventions

The third arm of treatment is the more invasive interventions, such as sympathetic blocks and nerve stimulators. Sympathetic blocks have long been used in the treatment of CRPS but the evidence of its effectiveness is lacking. One study found that only 50% of sympathetic block performed actually blocked the sympathetic chain.[41] Nerve stimulators also are used in the treatment of chronic pain. Spinal cord stimulators are the common stimulators used for chronic pain with one RCT demonstrating initial efficacy compared with physical therapy alone, but those gains diminished over time to nonsignificance at 5 years.[42]

Botox is an evolving tool in the treatment of pain. It blocks the acetylcholine release and this seems to reduce pain. It is being used intradermally to reduce pain with some early success and may be useful for cutaneous neuromas.[43]

Finally, it is important to consider peripheral nerve compression in patients with symptoms of CRPS. Placzek and colleagues[44] reported on 8 patients who developed CRPS following upper extremity surgery with clinical concerns for median or combined median and ulnar nerve compression, which were confirmed with electrodiagnostic studies. They were treated with nerve decompression, which resulted in statistically significant decrease in pain and increase in Disabilities of the Arm, Shoulder, and Hand (DASH) scores, with immediate relief of most other symptoms and improvement on motion and grip strength.

SURGICAL PATIENTS WITH CRPS

Management of a patient who has CRPS or chronic pain and may require additional surgical procedure can be challenging, as those with a history of CRPS are at risk for a recurrence/reactivation of their pain with additional trauma and thus this group is approached with caution. The first group of potential surgical candidates would be those patients with CRPS who also have a nerve injury, which is the pain generator. These patients include those with compression neuropathies or painful scar neuromas. Although there is no good evidence, most believe that surgery in this population is appropriate. For these patients, we first attempt conservative treatments (physical therapy, medication, rest, splinting, desensitization). If these fail, then we proceed with surgery. At surgery, we give our entire perioperative regimen, and if possible use an indwelling regional anesthetic catheter for the first few postoperative days. If possible, we limit immobilization and begin therapy shortly after surgery with the idea that it may be important to have the nerve gliding in the operative bed before scarring can tether or compress it. The second group is patients who might need surgery, but have had CRPS in the past. In general, this group should be approached with caution and unless the surgery has a high likelihood of improving quality of life, we would advise patients against surgical intervention.

Every practicing hand surgeon will see patients with chronic neuropathic pain and complex regional pain syndrome. There is much literature on these processes but most is in the anesthesia journals and not always readily accessible to the hand surgeon. We feel that the take-home messages are prevention for those at risk and that initiation of early treatment is something that hand surgeons should be comfortable performing.

REFERENCES

1. IASP Subcommittee on Taxonomy. Classification of chronic pain. Descriptions of chronic pain syndromes and definitions of pain terms. Pain Suppl 1986;3:S1–226.
2. Treede RD, Jensen TS, Campbell JN, et al. Redefinition of neuropathic pain and a grading system for clinical use: consensus statement on clinical and research diagnostic criteria. Neurology 2008;70: 1630–5.
3. Smith BH, Torrance N, Ferguson JA, et al. Towards a definition of refractory neuropathic pain for epidemiological research. An international Delphi survey of experts. BMC Neurol 2012;12:29.
4. Bennett MI. The LANSS Pain Scale: the Leeds assessment of neuropathic symptoms and signs. Pain 2001;92:147–57.
5. Haanpää M, Attal N, Backonja M, et al. NeuPSIG guidelines on neuropathic pain assessment. Pain 2011;152(1):14–27.
6. Evans J. Reflex sympathetic dystrophy. Surg Clin North Am 1946;26:780–90.
7. Available at: http://www.iasp-pain.org/Content/Nav igationMenu/Publications/FreeBooks/Classification_ of_Chronic_Pain/default.htm. Accessed February 5, 2013.
8. Harden RN, Oaklander AL, Burton AW, et al. Complex regional pain syndrome: practical diagnostic and treatment guidelines. Pain Med 2013;14(2): 180–229. http://dx.doi.org/10.1111/pme.12033.
9. de Mos M, de Bruijn AG, Huygen FJ, et al. The incidence of complex regional pain syndrome: a population-based study. Pain 2007;129(1–2):12–20.
10. Ciaramitaro P, Mondelli M, Logullo F, et al. Italian Network for Traumatic Neuropathies. Traumatic peripheral nerve injuries: epidemiological findings, neuropathic pain and quality of life in 158 patients. J Peripher Nerv Syst 2010;15(2):120–7. http://dx. doi.org/10.1111/j.1529-8027.2010.00260.x.
11. Boya H, Ozcan O, Oztekin HH. Long-term complications of open carpal tunnel release. Muscle Nerve 2008;38(5):1443–6.
12. Puchalski P, Zyluk A. Complex regional pain syndrome type 1 after fractures of the distal radius: a prospective study of the role of psychological factors. J Hand Surg Br 2005;30:574–80.
13. Kairaluoma PM, Bachmann MS, Rosenberg PH, et al. Preincisional paravertebral block reduces the prevalence of chronic pain after breast surgery. Anesth Analg 2006;103(3):703–8.
14. Obata H, Saito S, Fujita N, et al. Epidural block with mepivacaine before surgery reduces long-term post-thoracotomy pain. Can J Anaesth 1999; 46(12):1127–32.
15. Lavand'homme PM, Eisenach JC. Perioperative administration of the alpha2-adrenoceptor agonist clonidine at the site of nerve injury reduces the development of mechanical hypersensitivity and modulates local cytokine expression. Pain 2003; 105(1–2):247–54.
16. Zollinger PE, Tuinebreijer WE, Kreis RW, et al. Effect of vitamin C on frequency of reflex sympathetic dystrophy in wrist fractures: a randomized trial. Lancet 1999;354(9195):2025–8.
17. Zollinger PE, Tuinebreijer WE, Breederveld RS, et al. Can vitamin C prevent complex regional pain syndrome in patients with wrist fractures? A randomized, controlled, multicenter dose-response study. J Bone Joint Surg Am 2007;89(7):1424–31.
18. Besse JL, Gadeyne S, Galand-Desmé S, et al. Effect of vitamin C on prevention of complex regional pain syndrome type I in foot and ankle surgery. Foot Ankle Surg 2009;15(4):179–82.
19. Xie W, Strong JA, Meij JT, et al. Neuropathic pain: early spontaneous afferent activity is the trigger. Pain 2005;116(3):243–56.
20. Koh SM, Moate F, Grinsell D. Co-existing carpal tunnel syndrome in complex regional pain syndrome after hand trauma. J Hand Surg Eur Vol 2010;35(3): 228–31.
21. Grundberg AB, Reagan DS. Compression syndromes in reflex sympathetic dystrophy. J Hand Surg Am 1991;16(4):731–6.
22. Oerlemans HM, Oostendorp RA, de Boo T, et al. Traumatic peripheral nerve injuries: epidemiological findings, neuropathic pain and quality of life in 158 patients. J Peripher Nerv Syst 2010;15(2):120–7. http://dx.doi.org/10.1111/j.1529-8027.2010.00260.x.
23. Oerlemans HM, Oostendorp RA, de Boo T, et al. Adjuvant physical therapy versus occupational therapy in patients with reflex sympathetic dystrophy/ complex regional pain syndrome type I. Arch Phys Med Rehabil 2000;81(1):49–56.
24. Oerlemans HM, Oostendorp RA, de Boo T, et al. Pain and reduced mobility in complex regional pain syndrome I: outcome of a prospective randomized controlled clinical trial of adjuvant physical therapy versus occupational therapy. Pain 1999;83(1): 77–83.

25. Daly AE, Bialocerkowski AE. Does evidence support physiotherapy management of adult Complex Regional Pain Syndrome Type One? A systematic review. Eur J Pain 2009;13(4):339–53. http://dx.doi.org/10.1016/j.ejpain.2008.05.003.

26. Bowering KJ, O'Connell NE, Tabor A, et al. The effects of graded motor imagery and its components on chronic pain: a systematic review and meta-analysis. J Pain 2013;14(1):3–13. http://dx.doi.org/10.1016/j.jpain.2012.09.007.

27. Witt CM, Schützler L, Lüdtke R, et al. Patient characteristics and variation in treatment outcomes: which patients benefit most from acupuncture for chronic pain? Clin J Pain 2011;27(6):550–5. http://dx.doi.org/10.1097/AJP.0b013e31820dfbf5.

28. Christensen K, Jensen EM, Noer I. The reflex dystrophy syndrome response to treatment with systemic corticosteroids. Acta Chir Scand 1982;148(8):653–5.

29. Braus DF, Krauss JK, Strobel J. The shoulder-hand syndrome after stroke: a prospective clinical trial. Ann Neurol 1994;36(5):728–33.

30. Clarke H, Bonin RP, Orser BA, et al. The prevention of chronic postsurgical pain using gabapentin and pregabalin: a combined systematic review and meta-analysis. Anesth Analg 2012;115(2):428–42.

31. Maneuf YP, Luo ZD, Lee K. alpha2delta and the mechanism of action of gabapentin in the treatment of pain. Semin Cell Dev Biol 2006;17(5):565–70.

32. Moore RA, Wiffen PJ, Derry S, et al. Gabapentin for chronic neuropathic pain and fibromyalgia in adults. Cochrane Database Syst Rev 2011;(3):CD007938.

33. van de Vusse AC, Stomp-van den Berg SG, Kessels AH, et al. Randomised controlled trial of gabapentin in Complex Regional Pain Syndrome type 1 [ISRCTN84121379]. BMC Neurol 2004;4:13.

34. Varenna M, Adami S, Rossini M, et al. Treatment of complex regional pain syndrome type I with neridronate: a randomized, double-blind, placebo-controlled study. Rheumatology 2013;52(3):534–42.

35. Varenna M, Zucchi F, Ghiringhelli D, et al. Intravenous clodronate in the treatment of reflex sympathetic dystrophy syndrome. A randomized, double blind, placebo controlled study. J Rheumatol 2000;27:1477–83.

36. Fulfaro F, Casuccio A, Ticozzi C, et al. The role of bisphosphonates in the treatment of painful metastatic bone disease: a review of phase III trials. Pain 1998;78:157–69.

37. Tran de QH, Duong S, Finlayson RJ. Treatment of complex regional pain syndrome: a review of the evidence. Can J Anaesth 2010;57(2):149–66.

38. Saarto T, Wiffen PJ. Antidepressants for neuropathic pain. Cochrane Database Syst Rev 2007;(4):CD005454.

39. Kingsley WS. A critical review of controlled clinical trials for peripheral neuropathic pain and complex regional pain syndromes. Pain 1997;73(2):123–39.

40. Derry S, Lloyd R, Moore RA, et al. Topical capsaicin for chronic neuropathic pain in adults. Cochrane Database Syst Rev 2009;(4):CD007393.

41. Malmquist EL, Bengtsson M, Sorensen J. Efficacy of stellate ganglion block: a clinical study with bupivacaine. Reg Anesth 1992;17:340–7.

42. Kemler MA, de Vet HC, Barendse GA, et al. Effect of spinal cord stimulation for chronic complex regional pain syndrome Type I: five-year final follow-up of patients in a randomized controlled trial. J Neurosurg 2008;108(2):292–8. http://dx.doi.org/10.3171/JNS/2008/108/2/0292.

43. Ranoux D, Attal N, Morain F, et al. Botulinum toxin type A induces direct analgesic effects in chronic neuropathic pain. Ann Neurol 2008;64(3):274–83. http://dx.doi.org/10.1002/ana.21427.

44. Placzek JD, Boyer MI, Gelberman RH, et al. Nerve decompression for complex regional pain syndrome type II following upper extremity surgery. J Hand Surg Am 2005;30(1):69–74.

Management of Neuromas of the Upper Extremity

David M. Brogan, MD, MSc, Sanjeev Kakar, MD, MRCS*

KEYWORDS

• Neuroma • Management • Surgery

KEY POINTS

• Neuromas of the upper extremity are common, and their treatment can prove challenging. A multitude of operative and nonoperative techniques have been described with varying degrees of efficacy.
• Diagnosis of neuromas is based on physical examination findings and can be aided with the use of selective anesthetic injections.
• Several oral medications have been used in treating neuropathic pain, with anticonvulsants appearing to be the most efficacious.
• The underlying principle of all operative treatment is to remove the nerve or neuroma from any persistent source of mechanical irritation.
• Operative techniques can be divided into 4 categories: resection alone, resection with subsequent nerve grafting or primary repair, containment of the neuroma, or translocation of the nerve.
• The chosen method of treatment depends on the location and type of nerve as well as the injury sustained.

INTRODUCTION

After a nerve sustains a partial or complete injury, it possesses an intrinsic reparative capacity to establish continuity with its distal end. The ensuing proliferation of disorganized axons, myofibroblasts, endothelial cells, and Schwann cells can result in the formation of a neuroma (**Fig. 1**).[1,2] Reports of incidence range from 4% to 25%.[3–5]

Neuromas were first described by Odier in 1811,[1] with patients presenting with disabling pain or loss of motor function. Numerous treatments have been described, with varied success. In this article, the pathophysiology of neuromas, their clinical manifestations, and the role of current nonoperative and operative treatments are reviewed.

CAUSE AND PATHOPHYSIOLOGY OF NEUROMAS

The underlying cause of all neuroma formation is a degree of nerve irritation or injury (**Fig. 2**). Acute injuries are typically iatrogenic or traumatic. Examples of common iatrogenic injuries include damage to the superficial sensory branch of the radial nerve during dorsal exposures of the wrist or distal radius[6,7] or to the palmar cutaneous branch of the median nerve during carpal tunnel surgery.[8] Traumatic injuries generally result from lacerations to digits or the hand, which can result in stump neuromas. Subsequent repair of lacerations or replantation of digits with nerve repair can also result in neuroma formation, particularly if the segmental defect is long, excessive scarring occurs, or a mismatch in size exists between proximal and distal segments.[9]

When transected nerves are not repaired, end neuromas may result from fascicular overgrowth. When a nerve is injured or cut, signals travel retrograde through the proximal axon to the cell body to stimulate a reparative response.[10] There is a milieu of host signaling factors at the site of injury to direct the response, including substance P, calcitonin gene–related peptide, and mast cells,

Department of Orthopedic Surgery, Mayo Clinic, 200 First Street Southwest, Rochester, MN 55905, USA
* Corresponding author.
E-mail address: kakar.sanjeev@mayo.edu

Hand Clin 29 (2013) 409–420
http://dx.doi.org/10.1016/j.hcl.2013.04.007

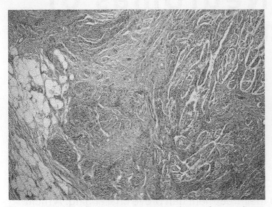

Fig. 1. Sciatic nerve neuroma resulting from above-knee amputation. (*From* Kitcat M, Hunter JE, Malata CM. Sciatic neuroma presenting forty years after above-knee amputation. Open Orthop J 2009;3:126.)

all of which may function to enhance the regenerative process.[11] Various neurotrophic factors, including neuropoietic cytokines, fibroblast growth factors, and neurotrophins, may also be involved. Within the distal segment, Schwann cells and macrophages begin to phagocytose myelin through the process of Wallerian degeneration.[12] The Schwann cells align themselves along the basal lamina of the distal segment to form bands of Bungner, which help to guide the regenerating proximal segment. This is accompanied by an upregulation of corresponding neurotrophic factors and neurite growth-promoting factors,[12] including neuropoietic cytokines, fibroblast growth factors, and neurotrophins.[13] Within the proximal segment, several sprouts form from the regenerating axon, each with a growth cone on its end that attempts to identify the suitable distal neural tube to guide regeneration.[14] When the regenerating unit cannot identify its corresponding distal segment, elongation cannot occur and an end neuroma forms (**Fig. 3**).[15]

Neuromas may also arise from crush or stretch injuries of the nerve, which remains in continuity.

Maintenance of the basal lamina allows for organized regeneration to distal targets,[12] but fascicular escape can still occur through disruption of the perineurium.[13] This subsequent spilling of the fascicles allows disorganized neuroma formation,[16] resulting in a neuroma in continuity.

Inflammation around a nerve can induce scar formation and accounts for a third mechanism of neuroma formation, even in the absence of direct neural injury. Scar tethering of nerves, or traction neuritis, results in activation of the nerve secondary to inflammation, irritation, or mechanical shearing.[17] Nerves of the upper extremity, specifically the digits, are at risk of mechanical irritation, given their proximity to the skin.

Despite their formation, not all neuromas develop painful symptoms.[2] Prediction of pain after partial or complete nerve transection is notoriously difficult, in part because of its multifactorial cause. Neuropathic pain is influenced by the presence of mechanical or chemical irritation, development of local scar tissue (ie, traction neuritis), and dysesthetic sensory symptoms.[1,13] In particular, proximal neuronal activity within the dorsal root ganglion, spawned by the injury, can contribute to the disabling dysesthetic pain. The type and size of nerve that is injured also influence the size and likelihood of neuroma formation. Injuries that occur more proximally lead to larger neuromas as a result of increased axoplasmic flow.[18] Nerves with a higher ratio of fascicles to epineurial tissue are more likely to form neuromas, because it is easier for the fasciculi to escape.[13]

DIAGNOSIS OF NEUROMAS

A history of sharp trauma, crush, or stretch injury along with a thorough physical examination can help diagnose neuromas. Pain related to a single peripheral nerve distribution, with or without accompanying numbness or diminished sensation, may also be useful in localizing the lesion. However, overlapping innervations of adjacent nerve

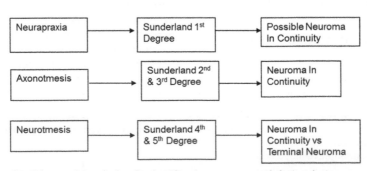

Fig. 2. Comparison of Seddon and Sunderland's classification systems and their relations to neuroma formation.

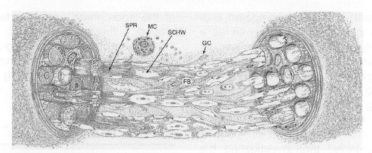

Fig. 3. Response of a nerve to complete transection. Sprouts (SPR) arise from the axons to form a regenerating unit, which has a growth cone (GC) at its leading edge. This growth cone attempts to attach to the bands of Bugner distally and minimize mismatch between axons. The zone of injury is filled with mast cells (MC), Schwann cells (SCHW), and macrophages. (*From* Lundborg G. A 25-year perspective of peripheral nerve surgery: evolving neuroscientific concepts and clinical significance. J Hand Surg Am 2000;25(3):394; with permission.)

territories can lead to some confusion when identifying the specific neuroma. Adjunctive measures, therefore, should be used to aid in the diagnosis.

Adjunctive Measures to Diagnose a Neuroma

- Tinel sign: The sensation of tingling when an injured nerve is stimulated via light percussion. This sign indicates the regeneration of axons and can be present in a nerve that is recovering or can be elicited from a terminal neuroma. An advancing Tinel sign distal to the site of injury is consistent with nerve recovery. A static or nonadvancing Tinel sign is more consistent with a terminal neuroma.[19]
- Anesthetic injection: Local anesthetic injections can help to pinpoint the cause when the diagnosis is questionable.[1] Complete resolution of the symptomatic pain or dysesthesias in the expected anatomic distribution of the injected nerve helps to confirm the diagnosis and show to the patient the expected area of anesthesia after neuroma resection, nerve transposition, or grafting.
- Imaging: Ultrasound guidance can be used to inject suspected neuromas when necessary to target sensory nerves located deep to muscle. Ernberg and colleagues[20] described the use of an ultrasound-guided steroid injection into a painful stump neuroma of the lower extremity, with complete long-term symptom resolution. If the diagnosis continues to remain uncertain or the clinical picture is confusing, advanced imaging such as high-field magnetic resonance imaging may be useful in these circumstances.

NONOPERATIVE TREATMENT OF NEUROMAS

Oral analgesics may have some efficacy in the medical management of neuropathic pain. The roles of antidepressants, anticonvulsants, opioids, and topical agents have all been investigated, at times with mixed results.[21]

- Antidepressants: In a randomized, double-blind, placebo-controlled trial of adults with spinal cord injury, amitriptyline was compared with gabapentin and diphenhydramine with regards to efficacy in controlling neuropathic pain.[22] In patients with high baseline depression scores, amitriptyline showed a significant difference in controlling pain when compared with placebo, but no difference was found in patients with lower baseline depression scores. Otto and colleagues[23] conducted a randomized, double-blind, placebo controlled trial examining the use of escitalopram, a selective serotonin reuptake inhibitor, in the treatment of polyneuropathy. The investigators found only a weak to moderate analgesic effect, with a 1-point reduction in pain on an 11-point scale.
- Opioids: Wilder-Smith and colleagues[24] compared the efficacy of tramadol and amitriptyline in a randomized, placebo-controlled trial of 94 treatment-naive patients with phantom limb pain from posttraumatic amputations. Initial complete relief of limb pain was seen in 67% of patients receiving tramadol, 83% of those receiving amitriptyline and only 3% of placebo patients.

Anticonvulsants

Anticonvulsants are commonly used in the management of neuropathic pain. Pregabalin and gabapentin bind to the α_2-δ subunit of calcium channels on neurons and reduce neurotransmitter release from synapses. A randomized double-blind clinical trial of 254 patients with neuropathic pain after trauma or surgery[25] showed a statistically significant decrease in pain scores for patients treated with pregabalin compared with placebo after an 8-week period, as well as a decrease in anxiety as measured by the Hospital Anxiety and Depression Scale. However, the overall difference in pain score between the treatment group and placebo was −0.62, on a scale of 0 to 10 ($P = .01$), showing only modest improvement and incomplete pain relief. Gordh and colleagues[26] conducted a multicenter randomized, double-blind, placebo-controlled trial investigating the use of gabapentin for the treatment of pain resulting from traumatic nerve injury. The primary end point for the study was the mean pain intensity score recorded on a visual analogue scale (VAS) from 0 to 100. There was a significant difference between the gabapentin group and placebo group with regards to change in mean pain intensity score from baseline to final week of treatment. However, patients taking gabapentin did note a significant difference in pain relief and improvement in sleep.

Adjuvant Treatment Methods

Before the development of oral pharmacologic interventions, several adjuvant treatment modalities were used for management of neuromas, including injection with phenol, alcohol, formalin and cerebrospinal fluid (of note, the last 2 are no longer practiced).[27,28]

- Phenol injections: Gruber and colleagues[29] injected 82 patients suffering from painful amputation stump neuromas with 0.8 mL of 80% phenol over 1 to 3 treatment sessions, resulting in complete initial eradication of pain in 15% of patients. Patients with lower extremity amputations and those with larger neuromas responded more favorably to phenol injections.
- Alcohol injections: Injections of alcohol into lower extremity stump neuromas has met with variable success. A series of 2 cases was reported in which 100% dehydrated alcohol was injected into the nerve proximal to the neuroma, with complete initial relief, and subsequent slight recurrence.[30]

Others have performed cryoablation, crushing, and cauterizing of nerve endings.[27] Desensitization therapy or splinting of the extremity may also give some symptomatic relief.

PRINCIPLES OF OPERATIVE TREATMENT OF NEUROMAS

When conservative measures fail and a suitable surgical candidate has been identified, selection of the appropriate operative technique centers around 4 therapeutic options: (1) resection of the neuroma; (2) use of nerve grafts to reconnect severed proximal and distal stumps; (3) containment of the neuroma; and (4) translocation of the nerve.

OPERATIVE TECHNIQUES
Resection of Neuromas

Neuroma excision is one of the earliest methods practiced. Tupper[31] reported the results of simple neurectomy in patients with painful postamputation neuromas in the hand and found that 65% had an excellent or satisfactory result. More recently, Guse and Moran[32] evaluated the outcomes of several surgical interventions in the treatment of hand and forearm neuromas in 56 patients, including nerve transposition into bone or muscle, simple excision, and nerve repair. Eleven patients underwent transposition of the neuroma into muscle or bone, 17 neuromas were excised without any additional procedure, and nerve repair was undertaken in the remaining 28 patients. Reoperation rates and mean Disabilities of the Arm, Shoulder and Hand (DASH) score were reported for each treatment group: nerve transposition, 36% (22.4); simple excision, 47% (31.9); nerve repair, 11% (11.4). Given the high rate of reoperation and poor resultant DASH scores, the investigators recommended against simple excision of upper extremity neuromas.

Despite these poor results, excision of a neuroma can be considered when certain criteria are met. These criteria include a palpable tender neuroma in the line of the damaged nerve, an inability to resect a neuroma and graft the nerve ends, persistent pain refractory to nonoperative treatment, and a neuroma adherent to neighboring muscle or tendons.[33]

Repair of Nerves

For digital neuromas in continuity, resection of the neuroma and use of a nerve graft or vein conduit to bridge the resultant gap may be used. Nunley and colleagues[34] reported on the use of a branch of the medial antebrachial cutaneous (MABC) nerve as an autologous graft for digital nerve repair, with modest success. Similarly, Malizos and colleagues[35] reported excellent relief of neuroma pain using vein conduits in the treatment of 23 patients presenting with 27 neglected lacerations or failed primary repairs of sensory nerves in the hand. Relief of the neuroma symptoms was achieved in 94% of patients, with return of good sensory function in 26% of patients and fair sensation in 43%.[35] These results were similar to a control group of 20 digital and 5 common digital nerves that underwent direct repair of nerve gaps within 1 week of injury.

Collagen tubes are gaining popularity to diminish postamputation neuroma formation. Thomsen and colleagues[36] reported on the use of collagen conduits in 10 patients with 11 digital posttraumatic neuromas in continuity. After an average of 11.8 months follow-up, none of the patients reported neuromalike symptoms, 5 of the 11 digits had good (6 - 10 mm) or excellent (<6 mm) return of 2-point discrimination, and the average Quick-DASH score was 19.3.

Containment of Neuromas

One of the most challenging problems with direct nerve repair or postamputation care is containment of fascicles from cut nerves, which may sprout into surrounding tissue, contributing to dysesthesias. Several techniques have been described to address this issue.

- Silicone caps: Tupper[31] described the use of silicone caps in 32 patients who had little relief with a simple neurectomy. Only 41% of patients obtained an excellent or satisfactory result. Swanson[37] reported a series of 18 patients with 38 upper extremity neuromas who underwent silicone capping as a revision procedure after previous failed neuroma surgeries. Fourteen neuromas (9 patients) had a residual Tinel sign postoperatively, but only 3 patients were dissatisfied with their postoperative results.
- Epineurial grafts: Epineurial grafts have been found to be more effective in minimizing postoperative pain as measured by VAS compared with epineurial ligature or epineurial flaps.[16] Results showed that the mean pain scores at 6 months were significantly lower for the stumps with epineurial grafts compared with epineurial ligature and epineurial flaps (2.06 vs 5.18 vs 4.25, respectively, $P<.05$).[16]
- Nerve capping; An autologous nerve graft is harvested and sewn to the distal end of the affected nerve after neuroma resection.[38] The distal portion of the graft is then left open, or alternatively, for fingers with both digital nerves amputated, a centrocentral nerve union is performed using a nerve graft.[39] Kon and Bloem noted an improvement in symptoms of 18 patients treated with this technique.[40] However, 7 patients continued to have tenderness to percussion at the site of the nerve union and 1 required reexploration at 6 months for recurrent neuroma formation.

Vein grafts may also be harvested and wrapped around nerves to minimize epineurial scarring in revision surgery or after neurolysis. Rat models have shown decreased scar formation after chronic nerve decompression with venous wrapping of nerves.[41] Clinical series using venous wrapping after revision nerve decompression procedures have shown clinical and electrophysiologic improvement[42] with minimal scar formation around the venous wrapped nerve.[43,44]

Nerve Translocation

Relocation of painful neuromas from the digits and palm into more proximal locations is a technique that has gained popularity.[27] The use of nerve relocation or muscle flaps to prevent or treat neuromas is based, in part, on studies that have shown that cut nerves form a cellular end cap when wrapped in innervated muscle, therefore decreasing neuroma formation.[45] In a primate model, Mackinnon and colleagues[45] showed that sensory nerves translocated proximally into muscle had less scar tissue than those left exposed near a wound or those retracted proximal to the wound.

For purposes of preoperative planning when considering nerve translocation, the hand and distal forearm can be divided into 3 zones,[46] each with their own preferred treatment strategy (**Fig. 4**, **Table 1**).

Zone I

Management options for neuromas in zone I include dorsal translocation and intraosseous implantation. Laborde[47] noted that dorsal translocation of symptomatic digital neuromas provided the most predictable relief in a series comparing patients who had undergone excision of the neuroma, ray amputation, neurorrhaphy, or translocation.

Boldrey[28] described intraosseous implantation in 1943. With this technique (**Fig. 5**), an end neuroma is mobilized and a drill hole placed through 1 of the phalangeal or metacarpal bones. Sutures are passed through the end of the nerve stump and passed through the drill hole to dock the nerve within the intraosseous space. Mass[48] described a series of 20 neuromas in 15 patients treated with this technique, with 14 neuromas in 11 patients showing good or excellent results.

Zone II

Zone II of the upper extremity encompasses the palm of the hand and includes, among others, the common digital nerves and the palmar cutaneous branch of the median nerve. Knowledge of these 2 neuromas is salient to the hand surgeon,

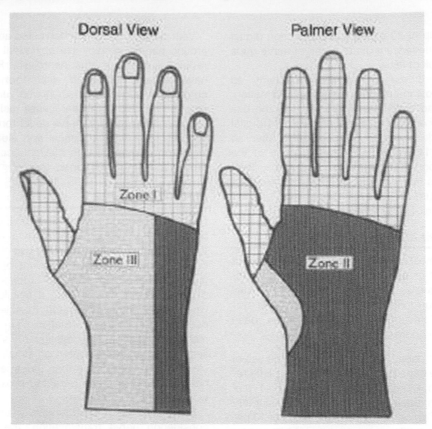

Fig. 4. Division of the hand and forearm into zones for planning of neuroma relocation. (*From* Atherton DD, Leong JC, Anand P, et al. Relocation of painful end neuromas and scarred nerves from the zone II territory of the hand. J Hand Surg Eur Vol 2007;32(1):39; with permission.)

Table 1
Neuromas of the hand and wrist and treatment options based on location

Zone	Nerves Involved	Relocation Options
I	Digital nerves	Proximal phalanx or metacarpal
II	Common digital nerves Palmer cutaneous branches of median and ulnar nerves Dorsal sensory branch of ulnar nerve	Pronator quadratus
III	Superficial branch of the radial nerve Lateral antebrachial cutaneous nerve Medial and posterior cutaneous nerves	Brachioradialis or other muscles of forearm

Adapted from Atherton DD, Leong JC, Anand P, et al. Relocation of painful end neuromas and scarred nerves from the zone II territory of the hand. J Hand Surg Eur Vol 2007;32(1):39; with permission.

because both of these may be injured during a carpal tunnel release, including the common digital branch to the third webspace.[49] If there is injury to the common digital nerve, Vernadakis and colleagues recommend neurolysis and transposition of the nerve between the superficial and deep flexor muscles.

Similarly, an approach to recalcitrant neuromas in continuity of the sensory branches of the median nerve of the palm is resection and grafting.[50] In this technique, the neuroma in continuity is visualized and the motor fascicles dissected out proximal and distal to the neuroma. The motor fascicles are preserved as a unit and the nonfunctioning sensory fascicles are resected and replaced with autologous graft (**Fig. 6**).

Atherton and colleagues[51] reported the results of 33 patients with 46 neuromas undergoing nerve relocation from zone II into pronator quadratus. Of the 46 nerves included in this study, 35 were relocated from the volar and dorsal palm of the hand (zone II) into the pronator quadratus. In cases of common digital nerve neuromas, internal neurolysis off the median or ulnar nerve was necessary to provide length for nerve transposition. The

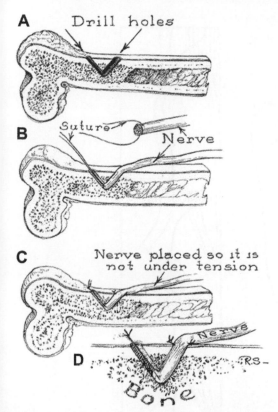

A Drill holes

B Suture   Nerve

C Nerve placed so it is not under tension

D Nerve   RS- Bone

Fig. 5. Original technique described by Boldrey for intraosseous implantation. (*From* Boldrey E. Amputation neuroma in nerves implanted in bone. Ann Surg 1943;118(6):1053; with permission.)

investigators noted that there was near-complete resolution of spontaneous pain and hypersensitivity at the primary site. However, approximately one-third of patients continued to experience persistent pressure and pain associated with movement at the relocation site.

For neuromas in continuity in the palm, Karev and Stahl[52] advocated mobilization of the lumbrical to serve as a volar pad and block to mechanical pressure. In a report of 2 cases with neuromas in continuity of the proximal digital nerve within the palm, the investigators describe a neurolysis, tenotomy of the adjacent lumbrical with palmar transposition over the nerve, and subsequent repair of the lumbrical. Both patients had excellent pain relief postoperatively, without any evidence of a Tinel sign.

Zone III
Historically, successful relocation of neuromas from zone III into forearm muscles has proved challenging in obtaining complete symptom relief, with patients often requiring multiple procedures. This situation may be in part because of overlapping innervation of 2 of the most commonly involved

nerves, the lateral antebrachial cutaneous (LABC) nerve and superficial branch of the radial nerve (SBRN)[53] and may require addressing both nerves at the same time. Elliott[17] recommends routine transfer of the LABC and SBRN together into the brachioradialis as the index procedure for neuropathic pain within this distribution, whereas Atherton and colleagues[53] advocate relocation of the SBRN into the brachioradialis, the LABC into the brachialis, and the MABC into the biceps.

Although these methods have shown promise when applied appropriately, success is not universal. Dellon and Mackinnon[54] analyzed a heterogeneous series of 78 neuromas of the distal forearm and hand treated with neuroma resection and muscle implantation. Overall, 42% had excellent relief of pain, 39% reported good pain relief, and 19% had little or no pain relief. Although the overall group of nerves encompassed neuromas from the brachial plexus distally, a total of 7 digital nerves were treated, with none achieving excellent results and only 14% achieving good results. Predictors of poor outcome after neuroma resection and muscle implantation included: (1) presence of a digital neuroma, (2) workmen's compensation; (3) 3 or more previous operations for neurogenic pain. In addition, patients who had nerve transfers into small or superficial recipient muscles, or muscles with large excursion, tended to have worse outcomes.

SPECIFIC NEUROMAS AND TREATMENT STRATEGIES
Pacinian Corpuscle Neuromas

Pacinian corpuscle neuromas, arising in the distal tips of fingers, can result after minor, repetitive trauma, such as sewing,[55] or from a singular traumatic event. Although the cause remains unclear, trauma to the digit has been implicated in 55% of reported cases.[56] Pacinian corpuscle neuromas are generally divided into 3 categories based on pathology: a single hypertrophied corpuscle, an increased number of normal-sized corpuscles, and an increased number of enlarged corpuscles.[56] Excision of the painful corpuscle is often successful, with confirmation of the diagnosis made histologically.

Bowler's Thumb

Initially described by Siegel,[57] bowler's thumb is a pathologic condition associated with repeated minor trauma to the ulnar digital nerve of the thumb.[58,59] This trauma leads to swelling and fibrosis of the nerve, resulting in a neuroma with altered sensation, a positive Tinel sign, and changes in 2-point discrimination on the ulnar side of the thumb. It is associated with bowlers

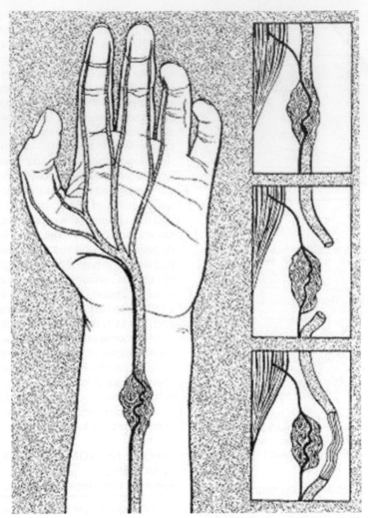

Fig. 6. A neuroma in continuity of the sensory branches of the median nerve with: (1) dissection of the sensory fascicles; (2) resection of the neuroma and preservation of the motor branches; and (3) grafting of the subsequent defect. (*From* Mackinnon SE, Glickman LT, Dagum A. A technique for the treatment of neuroma in-continuity. J Reconstr Microsurg 1992;8(5):380; with permission.)

because of the impingement of the bowling ball on the thumb and presents with a tender mass on the volar surface of the thumb. It can be treated conservatively with activity modification or equipment modification. Neurolysis, nerve transposition, and even neuroma resection have been used with varying degrees of success in several small case series and case reports (**Fig. 7**).[60,61]

Linscheid and Dobyns[61] described their experience in the management of 17 patients with bowler's thumb. Eight patients were treated successfully with nonoperative measures including the use of a plastic thumb guard or cessation of the aggravating activity, whereas 7 proceeded with surgery. Of these 7, 3 were treated by neurolysis alone, 1 underwent neurolysis and translocation of the nerve, 2 neuromas were resected and buried

in more proximal tissue and 1 neuroma was resected and the nerve primarily repaired. Six returned to bowling within 2 years, and the seventh was lost to follow-up. Swanson et al described a technique of translocating the ulnar digital nerve beneath the adductor pollicis. This required transection of the adductor pollicis and subsequent reattachment utilizing a suture anchor.[62]

Median Nerve Neuroma in Continuity

Median nerve neuromas in continuity can result from trauma or iatrogenic injury during carpal tunnel surgery. Dellon and Mackinnon[63] described the use of a pronator quadratus flap in the management of this condition. The pronator is approached from the radial and ulnar side and the

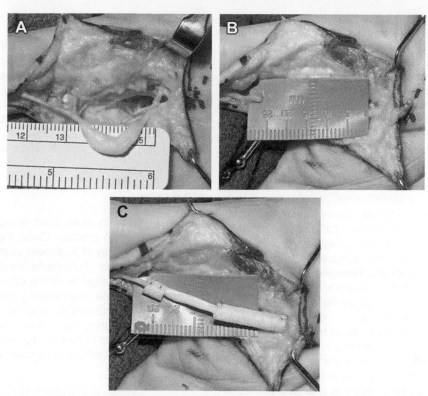

Fig. 7. Bowler's thumb. Examples of (*A*) neuroma in continuity; (*B*) resection; and (*C*) autologous nerve grafting and interposition of collagen conduit.

muscle detached from distal to proximal until the anterior interosseous artery is encountered. The muscle is then elevated with the pedicle and mobilized superficially. Given its limited excursion on the pedicle, it is best suited for median nerve lesions at the level of the wrist. In their series of 7 patients with 6 painful median nerves and 1 painful ulnar nerve, Dellon and Mackinnon[63] reported promising results in regards to symptom resolution. Six of the 7 patients had good or excellent results at 22 months after surgery, and the seventh patient's poor result was attributed to an injury to the forearm 6 months after surgery. De Smet[64] described a series of 4 patients with median nerve neuromas treated with pronator quadratus flaps; all were satisfied with their outcome and had improvement of pain, but mobility restrictions improved in only 2 of the 4 patients. Adani and colleagues[65] examined outcomes from a series of 9 patients over 5 years who underwent placement of pronator quadratus flaps over median nerve neuromas. Five of these patients had previous complete transections; the other 4 experienced partial transections, with all 8 undergoing primary repair and 1 receiving a sural nerve graft. All patients subsequently presented with wrist pain and a positive Tinel sign

over the median nerve and were treated with elevation of a pronator quadratus muscle flap to cover the median nerve. Of the 9 patients, 8 had pain relief and 6 had regression of their Tinel sign. None of the patients reported weakness with pronation.

Posterior Interosseous Nerve Neuroma

Neuroma of the posterior interosseous nerve (PIN)[66] is characterized by radiating, burning pain on the dorsal aspect of the wrist and hand. The diagnosis is confirmed with a local anesthetic injection into the PIN distribution. It may be associated with iatrogenic injury during ganglion excision and can be treated with PIN excision via a dorsal approach to the wrist.

In addition to the PIN, the superficial branch of the radial nerve can also contribute to burning paresthesias and pain in the dorsoradial distribution of the hand when injured. Neuromas in this area have historically been difficult to treat, and it is thought that the local anatomy may predispose the nerve to injury. Dellon describes how the nerve is tethered proximal to the wrist by adherence to structures underneath the brachioradialis. Any subsequent distal injury may tether the nerve at the wrist, predisposing it to mechanical irritation or shearing during normal wrist flexion and extension.[6,13] When treating these neuromas, relocation of the SBRN should be performed into the brachioradialis for optimal pain relief, because it has a small excursion compared with other local muscle options.[54] Attention should be paid to the possible contribution of the LABC nerve to dysesthesias in this region, potentially requiring further intervention for complete relief of pain.

MABC Neuroma

Neuromas of the MABC nerve[67] can be associated with iatrogenic injuries during cubital tunnel surgery. Treatment options for dealing with the resultant neuroma include conservative measures, as well as 2 possible surgical techniques, as described by Stahl and Rosenberg.[68] In their series, 3 of 12 patients underwent proximal resection, and 9 were treated by neurolysis, neuroma resection, and transposition of the nerve deep into the triceps muscle. Mixed results were noted in the former group, whereas in the latter cohort, good to excellent results were achieved in 8 of the 9 as defined by a postoperative VAS score of 3 and an increase in average grip strength from 55% to 87%.

INVESTIGATIONAL TREATMENTS AND FUTURE DIRECTIONS

Given that the formation of a neuroma results from an attempt by the nerve to heal the injured segment, some investigators have explored mechanisms to diminish the healing response. Bipolar and monopolar diathermy have been applied to the cut ends of sharply transected nerves in a rat model in an effort to minimize neuroma formation. This study showed a significant decrease in neuroma formation with the use of monopolar cautery for 4 or 10 seconds compared with the contralateral sharply transected peroneal nerve.[69] Bipolar cautery showed diminished rates of neuroma formation when applied for 10 seconds, but not when applied for 4 seconds. The investigators concluded that although diathermy appeared to lessen the rate of neuroma formation, the mechanism by which it is accomplished remained unclear.

Cryosurgery using a cryoprobe has shown promising results in a series of 6 patients who had failed conservative treatment.[70] Neuromas were explored at the time of surgery and left in continuity, with a 2 mm cryoprobe applied proximal to the neuroma or site of injury. The probe was applied for 2 minutes to freeze the tissue to −60°C, withdrawn for 30 seconds to allow the tissue to thaw and then

placed again for 2 minutes. All achieved good or excellent results postoperatively.

Investigations in animal models continue to look for mechanisms to diminish neuroma formation or mediate neuropathic pain. Crotoxin, a neurotoxin derived from rattlesnake venom, has shown efficacy in blocking pain transmission in a rat sciatic nerve model when the transected nerve stumps are immersed in the toxin.[71] However, the mechanism of this antinociceptive effect is still under investigation.

SUMMARY

Neuromas primarily arise from iatrogenic injury, trauma, or chronic irritation. Given their disabling symptoms, an array of treatment strategies exist, with varied results. Successful treatment relies on accurate identification of the offending nerve, containment of the regenerating fascicles, and cessation of mechanical or other noxious stimuli over the regenerating nerve end. The choice of treatment depends in part on the nerve affected, whether it involves critical or noncritical sensation, and its location.[49]

REFERENCES

1. Jaeger SH, Singer DI, Whitenack SH, et al. Nerve injury complications. Management of neurogenic pain syndromes. Hand Clin 1986;2(1):217–34.
2. Badalamente MA, Hurst LC, Ellstein J, et al. The pathobiology of human neuromas: an electron microscopic and biochemical study. J Hand Surg 1985;10(1):49–53.
3. Fisher GT, Boswick JA Jr. Neuroma formation following digital amputations. J Trauma 1983;23(2):136–42.
4. Lacoux PA, Crombie IK, Macrae WA. Pain in traumatic upper limb amputees in Sierra Leone. Pain 2002;99(1–2):309–12.
5. Geraghty TJ, Jones LE. Painful neuromata following upper limb amputation. Prosthet Orthot Int 1996;20(3):176–81.
6. Dellon AL, Mackinnon SE. Susceptibility of the superficial sensory branch of the radial nerve to form painful neuromas. J Hand Surg 1984;9(1):42–5.
7. Patel JC, Watson K, Joseph E, et al. Long-term complications of distal radius bone grafts. J Hand Surg Am 2003;28(5):784–8.
8. Louis DS, Greene TL, Noellert RC. Complications of carpal tunnel surgery. J Neurosurg 1985;62(3):352–6.
9. Meek MF, Coert JH, Robinson PH. Poor results after nerve grafting in the upper extremity: Quo vadis? Microsurgery 2005;25(5):396–402.
10. Wu J, Chiu DT. Painful neuromas: a review of treatment modalities. Ann Plast Surg 1999;43(6):661–7.

11. Zochodne DW, Theriault M, Sharkey KA, et al. Peptides and neuromas: calcitonin gene-related peptide, substance P, and mast cells in a mechanosensitive human sural neuroma. Muscle Nerve 1997;20(7):875–80.

12. Stoll G, Muller HW. Nerve injury, axonal degeneration and neural regeneration: basic insights. Brain Pathol 1999;9(2):313–25.

13. Watson J, Gonzalez M, Romero A, et al. Neuromas of the hand and upper extremity. J Hand Surg Am 2010;35(3):499–510.

14. Lundborg G. A 25-year perspective of peripheral nerve surgery: evolving neuroscientific concepts and clinical significance. J Hand Surg Am 2000; 25(3):391–414.

15. Maggi SP, Lowe JB 3rd, Mackinnon SE. Pathophysiology of nerve injury. Clin Plast Surg 2003;30(2): 109–26.

16. Yuksel F, Kislaoglu E, Durak N, et al. Prevention of painful neuromas by epineural ligatures, flaps and grafts. Br J Plast Surg 1997;50(3):182–5.

17. Elliot D, Sierakowski A. The surgical management of painful nerves of the upper limb: a unit perspective. J Hand Surg Eur Vol 2011;36(9):760–70.

18. Nath RK, Mackinnon SE. Management of neuromas in the hand. Hand Clin 1996;12(4):745–56.

19. Davis EN, Chung KC. The Tinel sign: a historical perspective. Plast Reconstr Surg 2004;114(2): 494–9.

20. Ernberg LA, Adler RS, Lane J. Ultrasound in the detection and treatment of a painful stump neuroma. Skeletal Radiol 2003;32(5):306–9.

21. Finnerup NB, Sindrup SH, Jensen TS. The evidence for pharmacological treatment of neuropathic pain. Pain 2010;150(3):573–81.

22. Rintala DH, Holmes SA, Courtade D, et al. Comparison of the effectiveness of amitriptyline and gabapentin on chronic neuropathic pain in persons with spinal cord injury. Arch Phys Med Rehabil 2007; 88(12):1547–60.

23. Otto M, Bach FW, Jensen TS, et al. Escitalopram in painful polyneuropathy: a randomized, placebo-controlled, cross-over trial. Pain 2008;139(2): 275–83.

24. Wilder-Smith CH, Hill LT, Laurent S. Postamputation pain and sensory changes in treatment-naive patients: characteristics and responses to treatment with tramadol, amitriptyline, and placebo. Anesthesiology 2005;103(3):619–28.

25. van Seventer R, Bach FW, Toth CC, et al. Pregabalin in the treatment of post-traumatic peripheral neuropathic pain: a randomized double-blind trial. Eur J Neurol 2010;17(8):1082–9.

26. Gordh TE, Stubhaug A, Jensen TS, et al. Gabapentin in traumatic nerve injury pain: a randomized, double-blind, placebo-controlled, cross-over, multi-center study. Pain 2008;138(2):255–66.

27. Herndon JH, Eaton RG, Littler JW. Management of painful neuromas in the hand. J Bone Joint Surg Am 1976;58(3):369–73.

28. Boldrey E. Amputation neuroma in nerves implanted in bone. Ann Surg 1943;118(6):1052–7.

29. Gruber H, Glodny B, Kopf H, et al. Practical experience with sonographically guided phenol instillation of stump neuroma: predictors of effects, success, and outcome. AJR Am J Roentgenol 2008;190(5):1263–9.

30. Lim KB, Kim YS, Kim JA. Sonographically guided alcohol injection in painful stump neuroma. Ann Rehabil Med 2012;36(3):404–8.

31. Tupper JW, Booth DM. Treatment of painful neuromas of sensory nerves in the hand: a comparison of traditional and newer methods. J Hand Surg Am 1976;1(2):144–51.

32. Guse DM, Moran SL. Outcomes of the surgical treatment of peripheral neuromas of the hand and forearm: a 25-year comparative outcome study. Ann Plast Surg 2012. [Epub ahead of print].

33. Birch R. Nerve repair. In: Hotchkiss RN, Wolfe SW, Kozin SH, et al, editors. Green's operative hand surgery. New York: Churchill Livingstone; 2011.

34. Nunley JA, Ugino MR, Goldner RD, et al. Use of the anterior branch of the medial antebrachial cutaneous nerve as a graft for the repair of defects of the digital nerve. J Bone Joint Surg Am 1989; 71(4):563–7.

35. Malizos KN, Dailiana ZH, Anastasiou EA, et al. Neuromas and gaps of sensory nerves of the hand: management using vein conduits. Am J Orthop 1997;26(7):481–5.

36. Thomsen L, Bellemere P, Loubersac T, et al. Treatment by collagen conduit of painful post-traumatic neuromas of the sensitive digital nerve: a retrospective study of 10 cases. Chir Main 2010;29(4): 255–62.

37. Swanson AB, Boeve NR, Lumsden RM. The prevention and treatment of amputation neuromata by silicone capping. J Hand Surg Am 1977;2(1):70–8.

38. Robbins TH. Nerve capping in the treatment of troublesome terminal neuromata. Br J Plast Surg 1986;39(2):239–40.

39. Gorkisch K, Boese-Landgraf J, Vaubel E. Treatment and prevention of amputation neuromas in hand surgery. Plast Reconstr Surg 1984;73(2):293–9.

40. Kon M, Bloem JJ. The treatment of amputation neuromas in fingers with a centrocentral nerve union. Ann Plast Surg 1987;18(6):506–10.

41. Xu J, Varitimidis SE, Fisher KJ, et al. The effect of wrapping scarred nerves with autogenous vein graft to treat recurrent chronic nerve compression. J Hand Surg Am 2000;25(1):93–103.

42. Varitimidis SE, Vardakas DG, Goebel F, et al. Treatment of recurrent compressive neuropathy of peripheral nerves in the upper extremity with an

autologous vein insulator. J Hand Surg Am 2001; 26(2):296–302.

43. Sarris IK, Sotereanos DG. Vein wrapping for recurrent median nerve compression. J Hand Surg Am 2004;4(3):189–94.

44. Vardakas DG, Varitimidis SE, Sotereanos DG. Findings of exploration of a vein-wrapped ulnar nerve: report of a case. J Hand Surg Am 2001;26(1):60–3.

45. Mackinnon SE, Dellon AL, Hudson AR, et al. Alteration of neuroma formation by manipulation of its microenvironment. Plast Reconstr Surg 1985;76(3): 345–53.

46. Sood MK, Elliot D. Treatment of painful neuromas of the hand and wrist by relocation into the pronator quadratus muscle. J Hand Surg 1998;23(2):214–9.

47. Laborde F, Marchand M, Leca F, et al. Surgical treatment of anomalous origin of the left coronary artery in infancy and childhood. Early and late results in 20 consecutive cases. J Thorac Cardiovasc Surg 1981;82(3):423–8.

48. Mass DP, Ciano MC, Tortosa R, et al. Treatment of painful hand neuromas by their transfer into bone. Plast Reconstr Surg 1984;74(2):182–5.

49. Vernadakis AJ, Koch H, Mackinnon SE. Management of neuromas. Clin Plast Surg 2003;30(2): 247–68, vii.

50. Mackinnon SE, Glickman LT, Dagum A. A technique for the treatment of neuroma in-continuity. Journal of reconstructive microsurgery 1992;8(5):379–83.

51. Atherton DD, Leong JC, Anand P, et al. Relocation of painful end neuromas and scarred nerves from the zone II territory of the hand. J Hand Surg Eur Vol 2007;32(1):38–44.

52. Karev A, Stahl S. Treatment of painful nerve lesions in the palm by "rerouting" of the digital nerve. J Hand Surg Am 1986;11(4):539–42.

53. Atherton DD, Fabre J, Anand P, et al. Relocation of painful neuromas in zone III of the hand and forearm. J Hand Surg Eur Vol 2008;33(2):155–62.

54. Dellon AL, Mackinnon SE. Treatment of the painful neuroma by neuroma resection and muscle implantation. Plast Reconstr Surg 1986;77(3):427–38.

55. Cho HH, Hong JS, Park SY, et al. Tender papule rising on the digit: pacinian neuroma should be considered in differential diagnosis. Int J Med Sci 2012;9(1):83–5.

56. Reznik M, Thiry A, Fridman V. Painful hyperplasia and hypertrophy of pacinian corpuscles in the hand: report of two cases with immunohistochemical and ultrastructural studies, and a review of the literature. Am J Dermatopathol 1998;20(2):203–7.

57. Siegel I. Bowling-thumb neuroma. In letters to the journal. JAMA 1965;192:263.

58. Marmor L. Bowler's thumb. J Trauma 1966;6(2): 282–4.

59. Howell E, Leach R. Bowler's thumb: perineural fibrosis of the digital nerve. J Bone Joint Surg Am 1970;52(2):379–81.

60. Dunham W, Haines G, Spring JM. Bowler's thumb: (ulnovolar neuroma of the thumb). Clin Orthop Relat Res 1972;83:99–101.

61. Dobyns JH, O'Brien ET, Linscheid RL, et al. Bowler's thumb: diagnosis and treatment. A review of seventeen cases. J Bone Joint Surg Am 1972; 54(4):751–5.

62. Swanson S, Macias LH, Smith AA. Treatment of bowler's neuroma with digital nerve translocation. Hand 2009;4(3):323–6.

63. Dellon AL, Mackinnon SE. The pronator quadratus muscle flap. J Hand Surg Am 1984;9(3):423–7.

64. De Smet L, De Nayer W, Van De Meulebroucke B, et al. Pronator quadratus muscle flap for the treatment of neuroma in continuity at the wrist. Acta Orthop Belg 1997;63(2):110–2.

65. Adani R, Tarallo L, Battiston B, et al. Management of neuromas in continuity of the median nerve with the pronator quadratus muscle flap. Ann Plast Surg 2002;48(1):35–40.

66. Loh YC, Stanley JK, Jari S, et al. Neuroma of the distal posterior interosseous nerve. A cause of iatrogenic wrist pain. J Bone Joint Surg Br 1998; 80(4):629–30.

67. Dellon AL, MacKinnon SE. Injury to the medial antebrachial cutaneous nerve during cubital tunnel surgery. J Hand Surg 1985;10(1):33–6.

68. Stahl S, Rosenberg N. Surgical treatment of painful neuroma in medial antebrachial cutaneous nerve. Ann Plast Surg 2002;48(2):154–8 [discussion: 158–60].

69. Tay SC, Teoh LC, Yong FC, et al. The prevention of neuroma formation by diathermy: an experimental study in the rat common peroneal nerve. Ann Acad Med Singapore 2005;34(5):362–8.

70. Davies E, Pounder D, Mansour S, et al. Cryosurgery for chronic injuries of the cutaneous nerve in the upper limb. Analysis of a new open technique. J Bone Joint Surg Br 2000;82(3):413–5.

71. Nogueira-Neto Fde S, Amorim RL, Brigatte P, et al. The analgesic effect of crotoxin on neuropathic pain is mediated by central muscarinic receptors and 5-lipoxygenase-derived mediators. Pharmacol Biochem Behav 2008;91(2):252–60.

Symptoms and Disability After Major Peripheral Nerve Injury

David Ring, MD, PhD

KEYWORDS

- Peripheral nerve injury • Coping strategy • Cognitive behavioral therapy • symptoms • Disability

KEY POINTS

- Major peripheral nerve injuries cause substantial impairment and highly variable symptoms and disability.
- As with other illnesses, the variations in symptoms and disability reflect mindset and circumstances.
- Given the substantial impact of these injuries, experts in physical adaptation and resilience (eg, hand therapists), emotional adaptation and resilience (eg, behavioral medicine specialists), and social and occupational roles (eg, social workers, financial advisors) are important members of the care team.
- Empathy and compassion aid recovery, even among patients with limited insight regarding the degree to which thoughts, emotions, and behaviors mediate symptoms and disability.

INTRODUCTION

Laceration and irrecoverable stretch, crush, or avulsion of a major peripheral nerve in the upper extremity causes substantial impairment in an adult patient. Radial nerve laceration causes the least impairment because the sensory deficit does not affect function (it is not on the finger pads) and the motor function (opening of the hand, which amounts to wrist, digit, and thumb extension) is usually restored with nerve repair or grafting, and can be also be restored with tendon transfers. The impairment associated with median nerve laceration can be more disabling than the impairment associated with ulnar nerve laceration because of the loss of the critical sensory function of the thumb and radial digits. Combined nerve lesions and brachial plexus lesions can cause even more impairment.

The substantial impairment of a major peripheral nerve injury is life altering. The recovery period is stressful and demanding. Reactive depression and anxiety are expected. Patients adapt, but it is difficult.

Hand care professionals who treat these patients encounter a wide range of coping strategies leading to varied courses of recovery and strikingly different final outcomes. There is evidence that the cognitive, emotional, and behavioral aspects of recovery (not to mention the circumstantial aspects such as worker compensation and litigation) are as important as the physical aspects.[1–3] Awareness of the factors that facilitate or hinder these aspects of recovery might improve the quality and effectiveness of our care.

DEFINITIONS

For the purposes of this article, a major peripheral nerve injury in the upper extremity is defined as an injury to any combined motor and sensory nerve resulting in substantial permanent impairment. Impairment is defined as pathophysiology, that is, an objectively measurable dysfunction in motion, strength, or sensation. Symptoms and disability are what a patient experiences as a result of the pathophysiology. Symptom intensity and the magnitude of disability are highly variable for

MGH Hand Service, Massachusetts General Hospital, Yawkey 2100, 55 Fruit Street, Boston, MA 02114, USA
E-mail address: dring@partners.org

Hand Clin 29 (2013) 421–425
http://dx.doi.org/10.1016/j.hcl.2013.04.008
0749-0712/13/$ – see front matter © 2013 Elsevier Inc. All rights reserved.

a given impairment and are strongly mediated by personal and circumstantial factors.[4] This is illustrated in the following example patients.

EXAMPLES

Guiding individual patients through the recovery process has brought these issues to life for me.

Patient 1

One of the patients I admired most was a nurse in her 30s who had an iatrogenic complete median nerve laceration during carpal tunnel release on her dominant right hand. When I met her about a month after the surgery, she was uncertain about her future. In addition to the pain from the surgical incision, she had the pain, numbness, and unsettling feeling associated with nerve injury and loss of sensation in the most important part of her dominant hand. She was trying to envision herself managing intravenous catheters and other daily job tasks and wondering if it would be possible. She was protective with motion exercises and hypersensitive, and her hand was stiff and swollen. I coached her on the normal human response to pain (which seems much stronger when there is an associated nerve injury), which makes us protect and prepare for the worst. I emphasized the importance of active finger motion exercises and use of the hand and assured her that although it definitely hurts, it is definitely safe and effective. She was able to change her mindset and improve her motion with little residual swelling, and we then proceeded with sural nerve grafting. She did well with her postoperative exercises. The hypersensitivity decreased over the next 4 to 6 months and she returned to work. She eventually regained slight palmar abduction and some 2-point discrimination. Despite severe residual impairment, she made good use of the hand, continued to work, and considered herself healthy. This bears emphasis. Her median nerve did not recover any better than average. She was numb and weak with substantial impairment of an important nerve. But she had limited pain and was able to do all the things that were important to her in a way that felt nearly normal to her. She was healthy despite a major change to her bodily function. She had limited symptoms and disability despite substantial impairment. Credit goes to her spirit, adaptation, and resiliency; not my knife or suture.

Patient 2

Early in my career, I met a man in his 80s who reported that his carpal tunnel syndrome (CTS) was much worse after carpal tunnel release (CTR). He presented about 4 months after surgery reporting that he could no longer position his thumb and his sensation was worse. The office notes before the surgery documented severe CTS on electrodiagnostic testing, with a nonrecordable distal sensory latency. The surgeon also documented thenar atrophy and severe weakness with palmar abduction. On examination he had no stiffness or swelling, a relatively inconspicuous scar, thenar atrophy, no palmar abduction, and equivocal sensation in the median nerve. I just could not get him focused enough for a good sensory examination. The story of an acute change was compelling and he was convinced that something went wrong so we planned surgery with Camitz transfer and possible nerve grafting. At surgery I found a narrow nerve under the transvere carpal ligament, but I cannot say for sure whether it was longstanding severe CTS or a cut nerve attempting to heal. I treated it like a lacerated nerve, placed nerve grafts, and did the Camitz transfer.

After recovery, he was happy with his thumb movement, unhappy with sensation, and could not keep from dwelling on the negative feelings associated with actual or perceived injury. I was so humbled and impressed by this patient that a few years later I studied the results of my CTRs and found that the most unhappy patients were those with severe CTS with atrophy, numbness, and weakness who were disappointed even after I explained that we could not recover those losses.[5] Some of those patients were disappointed with me personally and I did a few repeat surgeries with extended CTR until I felt more confident about the clinical scenario of operating on severe CTS and I got better (but not perfect!) at managing expectations. Now fewer patients are upset and even fewer consider repeat surgery.

This patient had severe impairment before his CTR. I do not think he appreciated how severe the impairment was. Looking back, he believes his thumb worked perfectly before surgery and his sensation was normal; unlikely given the objective electrodiagnostic testing. This patient's misconceptions led to what might have been an unnecessary surgery. Except for some thumb movement, it did not achieve his goals and he is still unhappy and unwell.

Consider at least 1 plausible way to construct his story that is very humbling. One year before seeing a surgeon for his CTS, we can assume he was severely impaired (numbness, atrophy, weakness) but he tells us that he had minimal symptoms or disability. He could depend on his hand and did not see it as a problem. At some point, he started looking at his hand differently. It is unlikely that the impairment and pathophysiology became acutely worse; that is atypical for CTS, which tends to worsen gradually over decades. So something in the way he perceived his hand changed. It changed enough for him to think that he needed to act. He needed to see a doctor and then a surgeon and have surgery.

The day he started perceiving the impairment in his hand as disabling, he set a goal that is unachievable for severe CTS. He wanted his sensation back. He probably found the results of surgery extremely disappointing. With the pressure off the nerve, it probably felt dysesthetic (what is referred to as "the blood rushing in" when a leg falls asleep and the pressure is taken off the sciatic nerve). Combined with the pain of the surgery and because he now noticed his inability to palmarly abduct his thumb (something that might have escaped his notice before), it probably felt like there was a surgical mishap.

Keep in mind that as this all evolves, there is little or no change in pathophysiology or impairment. And yet there are substantial changes in symptoms and disability. Enter a young hand surgeon as a second opinion, add a little stress contagion so that I also wonder if the nerve was cut, and in the context of such a long delay when interpreting the operative findings is equivocal, I may have been too aggressive and too hopeful that I had something to offer for return of sensation.

Although I explained that no matter what was causing the numbness (severe CTS vs laceration of the nerve) and my intervention had minimal chance of improving his function, we forged ahead. His impairment was slightly less with the Camitz and about the same in terms of sensation. His symptoms and disability persisted at a high level, still independent of the pathophysiology and much more closely tied with his mindset and interpretation of the symptoms.

Patient 3

A man in his 50s tried to commit suicide by swallowing poison and lacerating both of his wrists. I repaired partial lacerations of both median nerves. His spirits rapidly improved and he was good at his exercises despite the pain and numbness. He adapted well to the lack of palmar abduction of the thumb on one side (the other side maintained good palmar abduction) and returned to his passion for tennis in no time. Last I saw him about 1 year after the injury, he had permanent impairment of both median nerves, but made good use of both hands, was grateful, and considered himself healthy. Despite permanent impairment, he reported few symptoms and no disability.

Patient 4

A 30-year-old man had median nerve and brachial artery repair after a laceration on broken glass 8 years previously. His thumb and index finger were stiff in extension. When I coached him on stretching exercises, it seemed as if they were new to him and he flinched and vocalized with pain. We discussed reconstructive options. I told him surgery was not an option until he had full passive motion of the fingers and we arranged for coaching from our hand therapists. As we finalized our plans he requested opioid pain medication. He was cordial when I explained that it was against department policy to provide opioid pain medication for nonacute problems on a first visit. I never saw him again. It is safe to assume that he was looking for opioids and using his difficult problem to gain sympathy and perhaps fuel an addiction. It is important that patients and providers have shared goals that are achievable and that patients are prepared to do their part to optimize outcome. Major nerve injuries get our sympathy so systems and strict policies can ensure that we always do what is in the patient's best interest even if it is not what they request or hope for.

Patient 5

A pharmacist in his 50s came to see me for a phalanx fracture. I noted his near complete ulnar nerve deficit and we discussed it. The ulnar nerve was lacerated in the distal forearm by a broken intravenous bottle decades earlier. It was repaired, but recovered minimally. He had all the findings of a low ulnar nerve palsy. He had adapted to the impairment, never had any tendon transfers, and continued to work as a pharmacist. He was markedly impaired and minimally disabled.

Patient 6

A woman in her 40s came to see me after seeing about a dozen surgeons and having several surgeries. She had had an iatrogenic median nerve injury during CTR and had it repaired. She then had neurolysis followed by resection and grafting, followed by another neurolysis, followed by a vein wrap, and finished with a muscle flap. In the meantime she had also had cubital tunnel release and first dorsal compartment release. The symptom intensity and magnitude of disability were substantial. She was so protective, I could not undertake a good examination. She had atrophy of the thenar muscles, stiff fingers, and reported minimal sensation. We commiserated about the limits of modern medicine, reviewed the nonsurgical options and I never saw her again.

Compared with the other patients with the same impairment described earlier, this patient lacked the optimism, self-efficacy, adaptation, and resilience that help limit symptoms and disability despite major impairment. She continued to place all her hopes on external structural or medical interventions and none on the inner healing process. It can be argued that her marked symptoms and disability are due more to this missed opportunity for growing her confidence and self-efficacy than to the impaired nerve function.

Patient 7

A 55-year-old salesman injured his left nondominant wrist using a power saw to trim a tree. On presentation to my office, he had a complete median nerve laceration and a complex partially open and infected wound. After several debridements and parenteral antibiotics, the wound was clean and closed. The median nerve was repaired with sural nerve grafts. He was protective in response to the pain and dysesthesias, but meticulous and determined with his exercises. He regained full motion within 6 weeks. Two years after injury he has some palmar abduction and protective sensation. He is still troubled by the abnormal sensation and dysesthesias and has not incorporated and adapted to the permanent impairment of the hand. His focus remains on therapy, medication, and surgical options despite considering or testing every option. This patient is intermediate between some of the healthiest and most disabled patients I have described. In some aspects he has been adaptive and resilient, in others he has had a difficult time preparing for life with his impaired arm.

DATA

Cold intolerance, a symptom associated with many hand injuries but peripheral nerve injury in particular, correlates with disability.[6–8] Because reactions to cold vary substantially, at least 2 studies have tried to determine a cutoff on a scale that measures cold intolerance (Cold Intolerance Severity Scale).[9,10] One study chose a score greater than 30[9] and the other a score greater than 50 as abnormal,[10] illustrating the difficulty of determining a threshold of abnormality for a subjective experience that occurs on a continuum. Using the threshold score of 30, it was noted that 38% of people are cold intolerant after a hand fracture.[11] The same group noted that neuroma surgery could not improve cold tolerance.[12]

Several studies have demonstrated that major peripheral nerve injuries are disabling, brachial plexus injuries in particular, and that surgery offers slight improvements on average.[13–15] The work of MacKinnon and that of Novak and colleagues demonstrate other opportunities for increased health among patients with peripheral nerve dysfunction. A study of patients with nerve injury and nerve compression found that more than 60% of the variation in overall quality of life was explained by symptoms of depression.[1] A larger study of patients with nerve injury found that disability correlated more strongly with pain-related disability and illness intrusiveness more so than pain intensity.[2] A study of patients with brachial plexus injuries demonstrated that cold intolerance correlated more with disability and pain than with pain catastrophizing and posttraumatic stress.[3] A study of patients with peripheral nerve injury found that more severe injuries (brachial plexus) were associated with greater disability, but that work status, secondary gain, and pain catastrophizing were also important along with sex, pain intensity, time since injury, and age.

Given that subjective outcome measures such as disability/return to work, pain intensity, and cold intolerance are all measures of subjective aspects of the human response to pathophysiology, some correlation is expected. However, if the data on the psychological aspects of recovery from nerve injury were reanalyzed and disability, cold intolerance, work status, and pain intensity were considered to be response variables and were not also used as explanatory variables, it would probably be found that depression, catastrophic thinking, and secondary gain were as important or more important determinants of symptom intensity and magnitude of disability than injury factors (eg, brachial plexus and time since injury).

STRATEGIES

Patients with major peripheral nerve injuries need emotional support. It might be of value to screen patients for symptoms of depression and low self-efficacy (high catastrophic thinking). Patients with insight into how these aspects of the human illness experience create greater symptom intensity and disability could be referred for evidence-based treatments such as cognitive behavioral therapy.[4]

Given the substantial impact of these injuries, experts in physical adaptation and resilience (eg, hand therapists), emotional adaptation and resilience (eg, behavioral medicine specialists), and social and occupational roles (eg, social workers, financial advisors) are important members of the care team.

Patients who have difficulty seeing how mindset and circumstances affect symptoms and disability should be managed supportively with cognitive behavioral approaches in mind. Specifically, patients need help to understand that they will be able to adapt and make use of their hands, perhaps by putting them in touch with other patients who have made it through the recovery process. Careful choice of words and concepts is important to avoid reinforcing catastrophic thinking (eg, "work to pain and not beyond," "don't over do it"). Empathy and compassion are necessary to help them raise their spirits, inviting them to talk and tell their stories. Perhaps most importantly, placing hope only on medical and surgical interventions must be avoided, particularly if these might be based mostly on wishful thinking or they entail substantial risks.

Although treatment of these patients is time consuming and often not reimbursed well, the hand surgeon can have a substantial impact on the patient's recovery and well-being.

REFERENCES

1. Bailey R, Kaskutas V, Fox I, et al. Effect of upper extremity nerve damage on activity participation, pain, depression, and quality of life. J Hand Surg Am 2009;34(9):1682–8.

2. Novak CB, Anastakis DJ, Beaton DE, et al. Relationships among pain disability, pain intensity, illness intrusiveness, and upper extremity disability in patients with traumatic peripheral nerve injury. J Hand Surg Am 2010;35(10):1633–9.

3. Novak CB, Anastakis DJ, Beaton DE, et al. Cold intolerance after brachial plexus nerve injury. Hand (N Y) 2012;7(1):66–71.

4. Vranceanu AM, Barsky A, Ring D. Psychosocial aspects of disabling musculoskeletal pain. J Bone Joint Surg Am 2009;91(8):2014–8.

5. Lozano Calderon SA, Paiva A, Ring D. Patient satisfaction after open carpal tunnel release correlates with depression. J Hand Surg Am 2008;33(3):303–7.

6. Klocker J, Peter T, Pellegrini L, et al. Incidence and predisposing factors of cold intolerance after arterial repair in upper extremity injuries. J Vasc Surg 2012; 56(2):410–4.

7. Ruijs AC, Jaquet JB, van Riel WG, et al. Cold intolerance following median and ulnar nerve injuries: prognosis and predictors. J Hand Surg Eur Vol 2007;32(4):434–9.

8. Carlsson IK, Rosen B, Dahlin LB. Self-reported cold sensitivity in normal subjects and in patients with traumatic hand injuries or hand-arm vibration syndrome. BMC Musculoskelet Disord 2010;11:89.

9. Ruijs AC, Jaquet JB, Daanen HA, et al. Cold intolerance of the hand measured by the CISS questionnaire in a normative study population. J Hand Surg Br 2006;31(5):533–6.

10. Carlsson IK, Nilsson JA, Dahlin LB. Cut-off value for self-reported abnormal cold sensitivity and predictors for abnormality and severity in hand injuries. J Hand Surg Eur Vol 2010;35(5):409–16.

11. Nijhuis TH, Smits ES, Jaquet JB, et al. Prevalence and severity of cold intolerance in patients after hand fracture. J Hand Surg Eur Vol 2010;35(4): 306–11.

12. Stokvis A, Ruijs AC, van Neck JW, et al. Cold intolerance in surgically treated neuroma patients: a prospective follow-up study. J Hand Surg Am 2009; 34(9):1689–95.

13. Kretschmer T, Ihle S, Antoniadis G, et al. Patient satisfaction and disability after brachial plexus surgery. Neurosurgery 2009;65(Suppl 4):A189–96.

14. Liu Y, Lao J, Gao K, et al. Outcome of nerve transfers for traumatic complete brachial plexus avulsion: results of 28 patients by DASH and NRS questionnaires. J Hand Surg Eur Vol 2012; 37(5):413–21.

15. Dolan RT, Butler JS, Murphy SM, et al. Health-related quality of life and functional outcomes following nerve transfers for traumatic upper brachial plexus injuries. J Hand Surg Eur Vol 2012; 37(7):642–51.

Recurrent Carpal Tunnel Syndrome

Brian A. Mosier, MD[a], Thomas B. Hughes, MD[b],*

KEYWORDS

- Revision carpal tunnel surgery • Recurrent carpal tunnel syndrome • Median nerve

KEY POINTS

- In evaluating a patient for revision carpal tunnel surgery an important first step is to recognize whether the symptoms are persistent, recurrent or new.
- In cases of recurrent or persistent carpal tunnel syndrome the most common cause is a reconstituted or incompletely released transverse carpal ligament respectively.
- Though revision carpal tunnel surgery is technically demanding, patients will often have good clinical outcomes.

INTRODUCTION

Carpal tunnel syndrome is the most common peripheral nerve compression syndrome and the most frequent neurologic disorder of the hand. It was first described in the early nineteenth century, and has since become one of the most frequent surgeries performed on the upper extremity. The treatment of median nerve compression at the wrist has undergone progressive change over the years and has been successful at alleviating symptoms in most patients.

Complications and failures are reported to occur in 3% to 25% of cases.[1,2] Revision surgery for recurrent or persistent carpal tunnel is underestimated in terms of numbers performed and its technical difficulty.[3] Results following revision carpal tunnel surgery are disappointing, with up to 40% reported as unfavorable and up to 95% with persistent symptoms.[2] We provide a comprehensive review of the literature in the management of patients presenting with symptoms of median nerve compression at the wrist after undergoing carpal tunnel release.

CLINICAL PRESENTATION

The patient returning to the clinic after carpal tunnel release complaining of symptoms consistent with median nerve compression can be difficult to assess (**Table 1**). The patient's perception of symptoms preoperatively and postoperatively can be vague and inconsistent. A thorough history must be taken to evaluate for any new or undiagnosed disorders, such as hyperthyroidism, hypertension, or diabetes. In a retrospective review of 2357 patients treated with carpal tunnel release, 48 patients required secondary surgery and, among these patients, hypertension and diabetes were found to be significantly associated with carpal tunnel recurrence.[4]

The physician must discern whether the symptoms are persistent, recurrent, or entirely new. *Persistent* symptoms are those in which the patient never experienced any relief after the surgery. In contrast, the patient with *recurrent* carpal tunnel syndrome has an initial relief of symptoms after their index procedure, usually defined as about a 6-month interval. New symptoms are those

Funding Sources: None.
Conflict of Interest: None.
a Department of Orthopaedics, Allegheny General Hospital, 1307 Federal Street, 2nd Floor, Pittsburgh, PA 15212, USA; b Orthopedic Surgery, University of Pittsburgh School of Medicine, UPMC, 9104 Babcock Boulevard, Suite 5113, Pittsburgh, PA 15237, USA
* Corresponding author.
E-mail address: thughes424@aol.com

Hand Clin 29 (2013) 427–434
http://dx.doi.org/10.1016/j.hcl.2013.04.011
0749-0712/13/$ – see front matter © 2013 Elsevier Inc. All rights reserved.

hand.theclinics.com

Table 1
Recurrent carpal tunnel syndrome causes and treatments

Symptoms	Potential Causes	Treatment Options
Persistent	Incomplete release of the TLC	• Revision CTR

Recurrent	Circumferential fibrosis Reconstitution of the TLC	• Revision CTR
		• Neurolvsis
		• Interposition graft
		  ○ Synovial flap
		  ○ Muscle flap
		  ○ Hypothenar fat pad flap
		  ○ Vein wrap

New	Nerve injury	• Neurolysis • Nerve repair • Interposition graft

Abbreviations: CTR, carpal tunnel release; TLC, transverse carpal ligament.

symptoms that the patient did not have before the index procedure.[5]

Therefore, as a first step, it is important to delineate what the patient's symptoms were before the primary carpal tunnel release. The most common presenting symptom in primary carpal tunnel syndrome is intermittent impaired sensation in the median nerve distribution. Pain in the hand and wrist are the next most common symptoms, with nighttime paresthesias and weakness as other common complaints.[3] Patients with recurrent carpal tunnel syndrome often have the same complaints. In a retrospective review of 28 wrists in 23 patients with recurrent or persistent carpal tunnel syndrome, numbness was found in 27 wrists, numbness and tingling in 20 wrists, pain in 13 wrists, and weakness in 2 wrists.[6]

It is important, before primary carpal tunnel release, to document if numbness is constant or intermittent with exacerbations based on position or activity (ie, at night). These exacerbations are secondary to nerve ischemia, based on position and increased carpal tunnel pressures, whereas the constant numbness can be a combination of ischemia and chronic nerve changes. It is important to counsel the patient preoperatively that although the exacerbations (nighttime symptoms) may resolve immediately with the release of the transverse carpal ligament, the constant numbness may persist or have improvement over a prolonged period of time. With restoration of blood flow to the nerve and relief of the pressure within the carpal canal, these chronic nerve changes can improve over time and numbness may improve or resolve.

In those cases in which patients return for their first postoperative visit and report that they are "not any better," specific questioning of which symptoms persist is crucial to identifying the cause, and planning treatment for these persistent symptoms. Many will report that they still have numbness, but their night pain and dysesthesias have resolved. This suggests complete release of the ligament, and no immediate intervention is necessary. With observation, this numbness will continue to improve in most patients. It can be useful in these patients to perform Semmes-Weinstein testing at this point, as a baseline,[7] as this can be a sensitive method to monitor progressive nerve recovery.

Another unfortunate cause of persistent symptoms following carpal tunnel release is incorrect diagnosis. Often patients presenting with hand or wrist pain are erroneously given a diagnosis of carpal tunnel syndrome. This history combined with an abnormal nerve conduction velocity and/or electromyography may lead to surgery. Careful review of the symptoms before the carpal tunnel release, and afterward, in this population may demonstrate symptoms consistent with other hand pathology, such as stenosing tenosynovitis, carpo-metacarpal arthritis, or ulnar neuropathy. It is critical to elicit the history of symptoms before surgery to confirm that the initial diagnosis is correct and therefore treated appropriately.

When patients report persistent signs of intermittent nerve ischemia in the immediate postoperative period, greater concern is warranted. Concern over incomplete release of the ligament should prompt more vigilant follow-up or possible repeat surgery. Additionally, complaints of increasing symptoms should prompt concern over iatrogenic nerve injury. When patients complain of substantial postoperative pain, particularly dysesthesias, increased numbness, and demonstrate thenar dysfunction, the clinician should consider injury to the median nerve. To further investigate, the physician must explicitly define the time course of the symptom's development to distinguish between persistent or recurrent median nerve compression. The immediate onset of new symptoms after surgery, as compared with those that develop weeks or months later, is suggestive of an iatrogenic injury.

Initial improvement of preoperative symptoms, whether partial or complete, suggests complete release of the transverse carpal ligament. Delayed onset of symptoms following median nerve decompression, either similar to those experienced preoperatively or new symptoms (constant numbness rather than intermittent, positional numbness), are suggestive of scar formation or edema, causing restricted blood flow to the median nerve and resultant nerve dysfunction. In a retrospective review of 18 wrists in 17 patients with recurrent carpal tunnel syndrome, the average time between initial relief after the index procedure and the presentation of recurrent symptoms was 21 months, with a range of 7 months to 8 years.[1] In another retrospective review of 200 patients, the most common complaints of people who presented with recurrent carpal tunnel syndrome were numbness in the median nerve distribution and nighttime pain. The time between the index procedure and recurrence of a patient's symptoms ranged from 14 days to 3 years.[8]

CLINICAL EXAMINATION

The physical examination in the patient with recurrent or persistent carpal tunnel syndrome should be thorough and rule out other causes of nerve compression in the cervical spine and proximal sites in the upper extremity. Visual inspection and palpation of the previous incision should be performed and careful attention should be made to any tenderness elicited. Objective measures, such as grip strength or sensory testing, should be used when possible to quantify deficits in the affected hand. Provocative maneuvers, such as Tinel sign, Phalen test, and carpal tunnel compression test should be performed and compared with the contralateral side and with any preoperatively documented results, as up to 50% of patients with recurrent carpal tunnel syndrome have been reported to have positive Hoffman-Tinel and Phalen tests.[3] In addition, these patients experienced limitations in their ability to perform tasks requiring fine motor skills and had reduction in strength in the affected hand.[3] In another study of 28 wrists with recurrent or persistent carpal tunnel syndrome, 6 wrists had some degree of motor weakness and 11 wrists had some degree of sensory changes.[6] Tinel sign was present in 5, Phalen test was positive in 11, and Durken test was positive in 20.[6]

DIAGNOSTIC PROCEDURES

In addition to provocative examination maneuvers, the use of cortisone injections has been advocated in the diagnosis of recurrent carpal tunnel syndrome. In the context of a primary carpal tunnel release, it has been established in the literature that those who improved after the steroid injection had a statistically significant better response to surgery than those who did not.[9] The efficacy of the cortisone injection in recurrent carpal tunnel syndrome as a predictor of outcome is less clear. In Beck and colleagues'[6] retrospective review, the results of injection as a predictor of successful revision carpal tunnel release showed a positive trend, although they did not achieve statistical significance. This highlights the complexity of diagnosing recurrent carpal tunnel and, although individual positive physical examination test results and injections have not been shown to be predictive in terms of surgical outcome, they are useful when used in combination with other findings for diagnosis. In Jones and colleagues'[1] retrospective review, they found that a positive Phalen test, comparison of abductor pollicis brevis strength, and subjective splitting of the ring finger sensibility to be the most informative signs on physical examination. Beck and colleagues[6] used multivariate logistic regression analysis to combine multiple preoperative variables and found that when their model was adjusted for numbness and/or motor weakness in the median nerve distribution, a positive Durkan test, positive Phalen test, and relief from cortisone injection combined to provide a sensitivity of 100% and specificity of 80%.

As an adjunct to the physical examination, the use of electrophysiologic studies may be helpful. American Academy of Orthopedic Surgeons (AAOS) guidelines suggest that preoperative electrodiagnostic studies are a good practice in evaluating primary carpal tunnel syndrome. The use of electrodiagnostic studies in the context of recurrent carpal tunnel syndrome can be useful if the patient had preoperative studies done. If the repeated nerve conduction studies are worse or show signs of denervation of the thenar muscles, surgery is indicated.[1] In another study, the repeated nerve conduction studies were found to be pathologically increased, but there was no correlation between postoperative outcome and nerve latency or velocity.[3] This has also been confirmed in other studies in which the electrophysiologic examination after successful carpal tunnel decompression remained abnormal for up to 24 months postoperatively, demonstrating that it should not be used alone in diagnosis.[10] In contrast, improvement in conduction velocities indicates successful decompression and further surgery is generally not warranted. Interpretation of studies that are the same as preoperative studies is more challenging, and determination of treatment is less clear. Electrophysiologic studies can also be useful in localizing other sites of pathology.

The use of magnetic resonance imaging (MRI) or ultrasound has also been described, but the utility of these modalities has not been extensively studied and its use remains unclear. The AAOS guidelines recommend against the use of MRI in the routine evaluation of patients with carpal tunnel syndrome. Where MRI may be most useful is in helping to define pathologic anatomy when a benign tumor or other compressive entity may be suspected. Although rare, Stutz and colleagues[8] reported on 200 revision carpal tunnel surgeries, which had 4 cases (2 ganglions, 1 lipoma, and 1 fibroma) in which a mass was found in the carpal tunnel.

DIFFERENTIAL DIAGNOSIS

In most cases of recurrent and persistent carpal tunnel syndrome, the cause is incomplete release of the transverse carpal ligament, perineural fibrosis, or a combination of these 2 entities. In patients with entirely new or worsening symptoms occurring acutely, most of the literature supports injury to the nerve. This distinction is important in determining appropriate treatment.

For cases of persistent carpal tunnel syndrome, the most likely cause is either an incompletely released or reconstituted transverse carpal ligament. In Stutz and colleagues'[8] retrospective review, 108 of 200 patients who underwent revision carpal tunnel surgery were felt to have an incomplete transection of the transverse carpal ligament at the time of surgery.[8] Similarly, Jones and colleagues[1] reported incomplete release of the flexor retinaculum in 58% of patients. This study also demonstrated that the precise location of the incomplete release did not correlate with the original technique (endoscopic or open). For completeness, other diagnoses, such amyloidosis or an inflammatory disorder causing persistent proliferative tenosynovitis should be considered, as proliferative tenosynovitis has been shown to affect 7% of patients undergoing revision carpal tunnel.[1]

In recurrent carpal tunnel syndrome, the timing of the recurrence may play a role in identifying the etiology. In those who have rapid recurrence of carpal tunnel syndrome (<1 year) the likely culprit is perineural fibrosis causing traction injury due to spot welds or direct compression via circumferential encasement of the nerve. Renewed constriction of the median nerve in scar tissue causing tethering of the nerve has been found in 23% to 100% of revision cases for recurrence.[1,8] Other causes of recurrence include benign tumors, such as ganglions, lipomas, and fibromas.

Although scarring and perineural fibrosis are likely causes for early recurrence of symptoms, they are unlikely to play the same role in late recurrence (several years following the primary procedure). This is more likely a result of a recurrent increase in the carpal canal pressure. Following the initial release of the transverse carpal ligament, the ligament heals with a scar in an elongated position. As the patient ages, changes in the shape of the wrist due to arthritis and other degenerative conditions may lead to the increased pressures that cause median nerve symptoms. Although the etiologies are unknown, this is clearly a different process from someone who has recurrent numbness 6 months after a carpal tunnel release with initial relief of symptoms.

When a patient presents with new symptoms or worsening numbness, then nerve injury must be considered until proven otherwise. Certain patients may complain of trigger finger or incisional "pillar" pain as their new symptoms. These can be diagnosed by physical examination and require other courses of treatment. In patients with worsening numbness, with increased or absent 2-point discrimination, the physician should be concerned for iatrogenic injury to the median nerve. During revision surgery of the median nerve, iatrogenic injury was noted to have occurred in 3% to 6% of cases.[1,8] These injuries can be due to lacerations of the palmar cutaneous branch, recurrent motor branch, or digital nerve. Although rare, transection of the median nerve has been reported. Varitimidis and colleagues[11] reported on 24 wrists that had revision carpal tunnel release after endoscopic carpal tunnel surgery and reported that 1 patient had complete and 1 had partial transection of the median nerve. Another study reported 12 of 200 patients undergoing revision carpal tunnel surgery had iatrogenic nerve injury, with 2 complete transections. Both of these patients had undergone primary endoscopic carpal tunnel release.[8]

TREATMENT

When patients present with immediate postoperative symptoms and complaints of dense numbness, severe dysesthetic pain, and motor function loss, the treating physician should have high index of suspicion for an iatrogenic nerve injury. Although some patients with severe nerve compression can present with increasing pain from nerve reperfusion, this is uncommon. In these cases, strong consideration should be given to immediate nerve exploration. If there is doubt as to the severity of the nerve dysfunction postoperatively, a short period of observation may be warranted. However, if no improvement is noted in several weeks, exploration should follow. There is limited additional morbidity to exploration, but the benefits of early identification of an iatrogenic nerve injury and repair are substantial.

In most cases of recurrent carpal tunnel syndrome, conservative measures will not provide adequate relief.[11] Scar modification, splinting, and other exercises to promote nerve and tendon glide can be instituted. The limited ability to manage persistent symptoms in light of continued mechanical compression in instances of recurrence, whether by an incompletely released ligament, exuberant scar formation, or excessive swelling, means that in most cases, surgery will be necessary.

In patients with a significant interval between primary carpal tunnel release and recurrent symptoms, the authors typically treat recurrence with simple repeat carpal tunnel release. We define a "significant interval" as more than 1 year with resolution of carpal tunnel symptoms during this time. Studies have demonstrated good relief with repeat decompression at many time intervals,[6] and this seems most appropriate in these cases.

In patients who have a brief or partial improvement in carpal tunnel symptoms, or in whom classic carpal tunnel symptoms persist postoperatively, revision surgery is indicated. The revision carpal tunnel surgery begins by extending the previous incision into normal tissue to allow proximal or distal identification of the median nerve to first facilitate exploration. The transverse carpal ligament is explored. There is controversy regarding the extent to which the transverse carpal ligament can reconstitute and it is difficult for the surgeon performing the revision surgery to differentiate between an incompletely released ligament and a healed ligament. If the surgeon notes the presence of transverse fibers that are thought to be remaining or reconstituted flexor retinaculum, they are divided. The most likely fibers to be incompletely released are the most distal fibers of the transverse carpal ligament near the superficial palmar arch. The next most commonly identified site of persistent fibers are the more proximal transverse fibers or antebrachial fascia at the wrist crease.[1,8] The position of the nerve is usually radial and palmar within the canal. It is often adherent to the deep surface of the radial leaflet and can be associated with a severe perineural fibrosis. In most patients, this degree of circumferential fibrosis and scarring represents the most technically challenging part of the case when performing a neurolysis, as the nerve must be freed and mobilized from any scar tissue.

Following release of the ligament and neurolysis, a decision must be made whether to provide coverage in attempt to promote glide and minimize recurrent scar formation. The decision is often dependent on the nerve's mobility, position, and local soft tissues. If incomplete release of the ligament is felt to be the cause of the patient's symptoms, then no further treatment is needed and outcomes are expected to be similar to primary carpal tunnel decompression.[12]

When the physician feels that the local tissue environment is fibrotic and/or avascular, several procedures may be performed to help protect the nerve from recurrent scar, including autologous and synthetic nerve wraps and vascularized soft tissue coverage.

Other factors to consider are also ease by which the tissue can be obtained and the comorbidities associated with its harvest. There are generally 2 categories of these procedures, as explained by Azbug and colleagues[12]:

1. Interposition materials, such as vein grafts and synthetic devices to help prevent scar formation by providing a mechanical barrier.
2. Flaps that provide neovascularization, such as hypothenar fat pad flaps and synovial flaps, which can help to improve nerve regeneration and gliding.[12]

The ideal wrapping material should protect the nerve from compression by scar tissue, inhibit tissue adhesions to the nerve, improve gliding of the nerve during motion of the extremity, and decrease the scarring within the nerve trunk.[13] Synthetic devices used for revision carpal tunnel surgery have the advantage of decreased donor site morbidity, but at the expense of increased cost. Currently, there is not sufficient data to demonstrate they are better than autologous vein wraps.[12]

The vein wrap was initially performed in animal studies and demonstrated to preserve nerve function and organization by preventing epineural adhesion and restoring intrinsic epineural vascularity (**Fig. 1**).[14] More recent human histologic observations demonstrated that vein wrapping results in neovascularization without any evidence of inflammation and vein wrapping of the chronically compressed median nerve inhibited extrinsic epineural scar formation.[15] Furthermore, clinical evidence has demonstrated that patients with recalcitrant carpal tunnel syndrome who underwent revision with vein wrappings showed improved 2-point discrimination and electrodiagnostic findings.[12]

Pedicled flaps in revision carpal tunnel surgery are frequently used, as is demonstrated by Baratz and colleagues[16] review, whereby of 280 cases of recurrent carpal tunnel surgery 107 were treated with nerve decompression and flap placement, with pedicled flaps being favored over free-flaps. The hypothenar fat pad provides vascularized tissue to help prevent recurrent scar formation. The

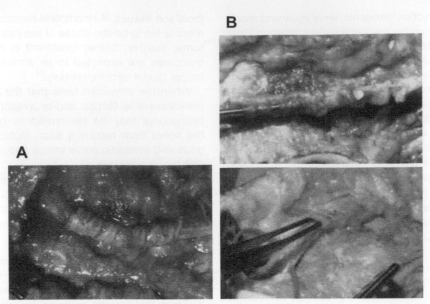

Fig. 1. (*A*) Example of a vein wrap used to prevent scarring around an ulnar nerve 2 years after being placed in a human subject. (*B*) Autogenous vein wrap with an instrument placed between the nerve and the intimal surface of the vein demonstrating that no adhesions existed. (*Courtesy of* Dean G. Sotereanos.)

fat pad, along with the ulnar artery, is mobilized and interposed between the nerve and the radial leaf of the transverse carpal ligament (**Fig. 2**). Strickland reported excellent results in 58 patients with 62 wrists who underwent revision carpal tunnel surgery using the hypothenar fat pad flap, with 37 of the 43 patients returning to their presurgery employment.[17] Craft and colleagues[18] reported on 28 patients who demonstrated improvements in 2-point discrimination and grip strength with 93% reporting less pain and 83% an improvement in numbness.

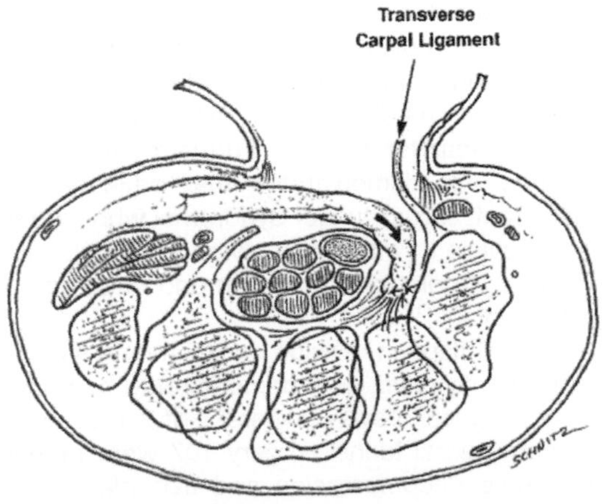

The synovial flap is a barrier to scar formation that is raised off of the superficial flexors deep to the median nerve (**Fig. 3**). The flap is raised and then sutured onto the radial leaflet of the transverse carpal ligament. The advantage of this flap is that the harvested tissue is easily accessible from the same incision and there may be less scar sensitivity when compared with the hypothenar fat pad flap. The outcomes, however, appear to be better with the hypothenar flap. Stutz and colleagues[10] compared clinical outcomes and electrophysiologic results of the hypothenar fat pad flap to the synovial flap, and the hypothenar flap appeared to produce superior clinical results, although conclusive statistical evaluation could not be accomplished.

There are no clinical studies comparing outcomes of wraps with flaps for revision carpal tunnel surgery.

CLINICAL OUTCOMES

The results of revision carpal tunnel surgery are variable, and many patients will experience some improvement but 41% to 90% of patients will report persistent symptoms.[7] There is little evidence to help the physician know what clinical features or diagnostic studies are helpful in predicting a good outcome after surgery. There are many variables, such as physiologic and anatomic factors, as well as psychosocial contexts, that can preclude a poor outcome. Some patients may

Transverse Carpal Ligament

Fig. 2. Illustration of the hypothenar fat pad flap with interposition of the graft between the radial leaflet and the median nerve.

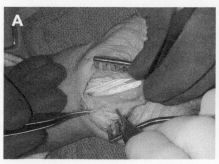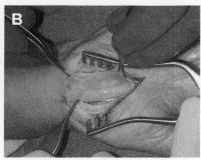

Fig. 3. (*A*) Synovial flap being elevated off of the FDS tendons. (*B*) Synovial flap before interposition placement on the median nerve. (*Courtesy of* Mark E. Baratz, MD.)

have improvement, but incomplete relief of symptoms after initial carpal tunnel surgery and the incomplete relief may prompt them to seek additional treatment. This dissatisfaction, in combination with a depressed mood, can confound symptoms and make it seem as though the situation is worsening, clouding the clinical evaluation.[19] It is commonly believed that other issues, such as workers' compensation claims, have worse outcomes. Beck and colleagues'[6] retrospective review of patients undergoing revision carpal tunnel surgery, however, did not find workers' compensation status to be a predictor of outcomes. In their review, gender, age, hand dominance, history of smoking or trauma, numbness/tingling, weakness, and pain all failed to be statistically significant predictors of surgical outcome. Intraoperative findings that have been shown to have poorer outcomes are severe circumferential fibrosis around the median nerve, proliferative tenosynovitis, and amyloidosis.[1] The outcome ultimately lies with the pathology causing mechanical compression. Patients with an incompletely released transverse ligament can expect to have outcomes similar to primary carpal tunnel release. In more severe cases with circumferential fibrosis causing decreased vascularity or traction injury to the median nerve, outcomes are less predictable. Although there are no prospective data differentiating which treatment algorithm is the best for recurrent carpal tunnel, there is a trend in the literature toward favoring vascularized coverage with flaps, with the hypothenar fat pad flap appearing to have equal or better results than the others in clinical results and electrophysiologic testing.[2,10]

SUMMARY

Recurrent carpal tunnel syndrome is difficult to diagnose and treat. The clinical examination and workup after primary carpal tunnel surgery can

be confusing and fraught with a number of confounding variables. In patients with persistent or recurrent symptoms, exploration with repeat transverse carpal ligament release and median nerve neurolysis may be performed. If severe scarring is noted, the use of an interposition material or flap is warranted. If the patient presents with new or worsening symptoms of numbness or weakness after carpal tunnel surgery, then the physician must be concerned for iatrogenic nerve injury and exploration with repair should be considered. Although patients may not obtain complete relief of symptoms as readily as after primary carpal tunnel release, the literature supports repeat surgery, as improvement often occurs.

REFERENCES

1. Jones N, Ahn CH, Eo S. Revision surgery for persistent and recurrent carpal tunnel syndrome and for failed carpal tunnel release. Plast Reconstr Surg 2012;129:683–92.
2. Tollestrup T, Berg C, Netscher D. Management of distal traumatic median nerve painful neuromas and of recurrent carpal tunnel syndrome: hypothenar fat pad flap. J Hand Surg Am 2010;35: 1010–4.
3. Unglaub F, Wolf E, Goldbach C. Subjective and functional outcome after revision surgery in carpal tunnel syndrome. Arch Orthop Trauma Surg 2008; 128:931–6.
4. Schreiber JE, Foran MP, Schreiber DJ, et al. Common risk factors seen in secondary carpal tunnel surgery. Ann Plast Surg 2005;55:262–5.
5. Tung TH, Mackinnon SE. Secondary carpal tunnel surgery. Plast Reconstr Surg 2001;107:1830–43 [quiz: 1844–933].
6. Beck J, Brothers J, Maloney P. Predicting the outcome of revision carpal tunnel release. J Hand Surg Am 2012;37:282–7.
7. Steyers C. Recurrent carpal tunnel syndrome. Hand Clin 2002;18:339–45.

8. Stutz N, Gohritz A, Van Schoonhoven J. Revision surgery after carpal tunnel release analysis of the pathology in 200 cases during a 2 year period. J Hand Surg Br 2006;31:68–71.

9. Edgell SE, McCabe SJ, Breidenbach WC. Predicting the outcome of carpal tunnel release. J Hand Surg Am 2003;28:255–61.

10. Stutz N, Gohritz A, Novotny A. Clinical and electrophysiological comparison of different methods of soft tissue coverage of the median nerve in recurrent carpal tunnel syndrome. Neurosurgery 2008;62:194–8.

11. Varitimidis S, Herndon J, Sotereanos D. Failed endoscopic carpal tunnel release. J Hand Surg Br 1999; 24:465–7.

12. Azbug J, Jacoby S, Osterman A. Surgical options for recalcitrant carpal tunnel syndrome with perineural fibrosis. Hand 2012;7:23–9.

13. Sarris I, Sotereanos D. Vein wrapping for recurrent median nerve compression. Hand 2004;4:189–94.

14. Xu J, Varitimidis SE, Fisher KJ, et al. The effect of wrapping scarred nerves with autogenous graft to treat recurrent chronic nerve compression. J Hand Surg Am 2000;25:93–103.

15. Chou K, Papadimitriou NG, Sarris I. Neovascularization and other histopathologic findings in an autogenous saphenous vein wrap used for recalcitrant carpal tunnel syndrome: a case report. J Hand Surg Am 2003;28:262–6.

16. Gannon C, Baratz K, Baratz M. The synovial flap in recurrent and failed carpal tunnel surgery. Oper Tech Orthop 2007;17:102–5.

17. Strickland JW, Idler RS, Lourie GM, et al. The hypothenar fat pad flap for management of recalcitrant carpal tunnel syndrome. J Hand Surg Am 1996;21: 840–8.

18. Craft RO, Duncan SF, Smith A. Management of recurrent carpal tunnel syndrome with microlysis and the hypothenar fat pad flap. Hand 2007;2: 85–9.

19. Amadio P. Interventions for recurrent/persistent carpal tunnel syndrome after carpal tunnel release. Hand 2009;34:1320–2.

Ulnar Neuropathy at the Elbow
An Evidence-based Algorithm

Peter C. Chimenti, MD, Warren C. Hammert, MD*

KEYWORDS

- Ulnar neuropathy • Cubital tunnel syndrome • Ulnar nerve • Nerve transposition • Endoscopic
- Nerve compression

KEY POINTS

- Current evidence suggests that the different surgical methods to treat UNE do not differ in their clinical outcomes.
- Lack of standardized grading systems and outcome measures makes preoperatively determining of which type of procedure to perform impossible at this time.
- Outcomes for revision surgery are poorer than primary procedures.
- Anterior transposition is commonly used for revision cases but no literature is available to support this practice.

INTRODUCTION

From its origin at the brachial plexus to entering Guyon canal at the wrist, the ulnar nerve may be compressed at multiple levels; however, the cubital tunnel represents the most common site of compression and the target of numerous surgical techniques that are aimed at decompressing and/or relieving tension on the nerve at this level.[1–3] The aim of this review is to discuss current literature on clinical and functional outcomes after surgical treatment of ulnar neuropathy at the elbow (UNE), focusing on the best available evidence. As the methodological quality of orthopedic research continues to improve from retrospective case series to prospective randomized clinical trials (RCT), the goal of developing an evidence-based algorithm to guide clinical decision making hopefully may be reached.

PATHOPHYSIOLOGY

With progressive elbow flexion, the ulnar nerve experiences friction, traction, and compression forces.[2,4] In a cadaver study, Gelberman and colleagues[5] advocated that traction is responsible for the increase in intraneural pressure found with progressive elbow flexion to 130°. Wright and colleagues[6] demonstrated unrestricted upper extremity motion could produce up to a 29% increase in ulnar nerve length, placing substantial strain on the nerve. Several sites of compression are possible, including the medial intramuscular septum, the internal brachial ligament, the cubital tunnel, and the flexor-pronator aponeurosis. Although compression most commonly occurs at the level of the cubital tunnel,[3] it is important to realize that both the fibrous canal located 7 cm to 8 cm proximal to the epicondyle as well as fibrous bands within the flexor carpi ulnaris[7] are additional potential sites of compression, and decompression at these sites should be strongly considered to prevent incomplete release of the ulnar nerve. Less common sources of compression include osteophytes from degenerative arthritis, tumors, vascular malformations, anomalous bands of fibrous tissue, and the anconeus epitrochlearis muscle.[1] Anterior transposition should eliminate both pathologic traction and compression forces on the nerve[8]; however, extensive mobilization

Department of Orthopaedics, University of Rochester Medical Center, 601 Elmwood Avenue, Box 665, Rochester, NY 14642, USA
* Corresponding author.
E-mail address: Warren_Hammert@urmc.rochester.edu

Hand Clin 29 (2013) 435–442
http://dx.doi.org/10.1016/j.hcl.2013.04.013
0749-0712/13/$ – see front matter © 2013 Elsevier Inc. All rights reserved.

necessary for transposition has the potential for segmental transient devascularization, which may exacerbate the problem.[9] Proponents of transposition have argued that in situ decompression fails to address hypermobility and may, therefore, be unsuccessful. It remains unclear, however, whether or not preoperative or intraoperative nerve subluxation is correlated with clinical outcomes.

STAGING SYSTEMS AND OUTCOME MEASURES

Several classification systems of UNE severity have been proposed. In 1950, McGowan[10,11] described a subjective system that is still routinely used (Table 1). In 1989, Dellon[12] introduced his classification that scores patients on a 10-point numeric scale based on objective physical findings, including 2-point discrimination and vibratory perception, muscle weakness, and atrophy. Subjective outcomes are important in determining the effectiveness of treatment. Unfortunately, subjective outcomes for treatment of UNE lag behind those for carpal tunnel syndrome.[13] The most widely used outcome measure was reported by Wilson and Krout in 1973[14] and qualitatively divided patient outcomes from excellent to poor. Macadam and colleagues[15] performed a systematic review looking at outcome measures for UNE that identified 13 reports of unique author-generated scales and found that most studies report outcomes as excellent/good/fair/poor. Only 1 study to date has reported a validated, patient-based measure to assess symptoms.[16] In 2006, Mondelli and colleagues described a 9-item questionnaire, the UNE questionnaire, which focuses primarily on numbness and tingling in the small and ring fingers, elbow pain, and change in symptoms with elbow positioning.

In addition to generic quality-of-life measures, such as the 36-Item Short Form Health Survey and visual analogue scale (VAS), upper extremity specific measures, such as the Disability of the Arm, Shoulder and Hand Questionnaire, have been used to describe outcomes, but impairment resulting from UNE is often not severe enough to create a meaningful change in these more general measures of overall or upper extremity health.

EXAMINING THE LITERATURE

In 1998, Bartels and colleagues[17] performed a systematic review of the literature from 1970 through 1997, including all levels of evidence available. Statistical combination of the studies was performed by grading the preoperative and postoperative McGowan classification grades, which resulted in more than 2000 patients; however, only 2 of the included studies were prospective and none was a RCT. When analyzed in relation to their preoperative McGowan classification grade, those patients with grade 1 or 2 had the best outcomes from in situ decompression whereas the more severely affected grade 3 patients had better results with anterior intramuscular transposition. The investigators suggested that in situ release be performed initially in all patients along with an intraoperative assessment of nerve stability and subsequent transposition only for those nerves that sublux with elbow flexion. Using this study as a starting point, this article reviews the subsequent literature on clinical and functional outcomes.

In Situ Release

Karthik and colleagues[18] published on a prospective cohort of 30 patients with severe ulnar neuropathy undergoing simple decompression using a minimally invasive approach (<4 cm incision) (level III); 80% good to excellent results were noted at 1 year without any complications. Pavelka and colleagues[19] retrospectively examined 55 patients at 13 months; 70% were Dellon grade 3 preoperatively and 80% were very satisfied with their outcome (level IV). Long-term outcomes suggest that approximately 62% of patients show substantial subjective improvement between 1-year and 12-year follow-up[20] (level IV). Taniguchi and coworkers[21] used a minimally invasive approach (2-cm longitudinal incision) for simple decompression in their study of 18 patients retrospectively examined at 14 months (level IV). These investigators report 77% good to excellent results and only

Table 1
McGowan classification of ulnar neuropathy at the elbow, as modified by Goldberg

Grade	Sensory Symptoms	Motor Examination
1	Mild parasthesias or sensory loss	No weakness
2A	Moderate sensory loss	No intrinsic atrophy, mild weakness
2B	Moderate sensory loss	3/5 Intrinsic strength, moderate weakness
3	Severe sensory loss or parasthesias	Severe intrinsic atrophy and weakness

Data from Goldberg BJ, Light TR, Blair SJ. Ulnar neuropathy at the elbow: results of medial epicondylectomy. J Hand Surg Am 1989;14(2 Pt 1):182–8.

1 case of postoperative hematoma not requiring reoperation. Together these studies suggest 60% to 90% good to excellent outcomes with a trend toward better outcomes for less-severe preoperative grades.

Medial Epicondylectomy

Medial epicondylectomy seeks to relieve strain on the nerve by allowing it to glide anteriorly and may be performed as a partial (>40%) or minimal (<20%) resection of the epicondyle with or without decompression. Concerns regarding postoperative nerve subluxation, valgus elbow instability, and bony tenderness have been reported.[9] The authors were not able to identify any studies with higher levels of evidence (level I/II) for medial epicondylectomy. Existing literature includes retrospective outcomes or comparative cohort studies.[22–26] Using the Wilson/Krout criteria, reported outcomes among the retrospective case series are similar, with 75% to 79% good to excellent results[23,25] even among patients with the most severe disease.[24] Amako and colleagues[22] retrospectively compared partial (40%–80% resection) and minimal medial epicondylectomy (<20%) and found no difference in clinical or neurophysiologic outcomes between the groups but reported a 74% rate of valgus instability in the partial cohort compared with 0% in the minimal cohort group (level III). Pain over the osteotomy site is reported, with rates between 13% and 45% at 6 months to 3 years. Complications or adverse events reported with this procedure include medial elbow dysesthesias due to injury to branches of the medial antebrachial cutaneous (MABC) nerve (7%), revision to submuscular transposition (7%), and painful subluxation (13%).[25] Seradge defined recurrence as return of symptoms after 3 months of clinical improvement and reported a rate of 13% at 3 years[26] (level III).

Anterior Transposition

After anterior transposition, the ulnar nerve may be placed in a subcutaneous, intramuscular, or submuscular location, with the latter requiring the most extensive dissection.[3] Transposition procedures are commonly used for revision surgery or more severe stages of neuropathy based on the concept that transposition relieves tension more than in situ decompression or medial epicondylectomy. Some investigators argue that the amount of soft tissue dissection necessary may increase the risk of postoperative infection or recurrence from scar tissue formation.[9,27] After subcutaneous anterior transposition, good to excellent results

have been reported in 84% to 94% of cases in level IV retrospective case series.[28–30]

In a prospective cohort study of 29 patients undergoing subcutaneous transposition, Hamidreza and colleagues[31] noted 62% good to excellent results at 1 month, increasing to 82% at 12 months, as well as a correlation between preoperative grade and postoperative outcome with an odds ratio of 3 for fair or poor outcome in the most severe cases (level III). Iba and colleagues[32] noted that patients undergoing subcutaneous transposition who have osteoarthritis at the elbow with osteophytes in the cubital tunnel might require a more extensive release to achieve good outcomes (level III). Several reports suggest that injury to branches of the MABC during dissection is a potential complication of transposition.[33–35] Fitzgerald and colleagues[34] reported 19 of 20 patients had excellent results 2 years after submuscular transposition, with 2 transient and 1 permanent MABC neurapraxias (level IV).

At least 2 studies comparing different transposition techniques have failed to show subtantial differences in clinical outcomes.[36,37] Charles and colleagues[36] reported similar motor and sensory recovery in patients with moderate and severe disease treated with either submuscular or subcutaneous anterior transposition in a retrospective case comparison (level III). In a similarly designed study, Kose and colleagues[37] retrospectively reviewed patients who underwent anterior transposition to subcutaneous, submuscular, or intramuscular position and reported an overall rate of 77% good to excellent results and a trend toward less improvement among McGowan grade 3 patients (level III).

In an attempt to predict preoperative factors that may affect postoperative outcome for all types of transposition, Shi and colleagues[38] performed a systematic review of the literature (level III). The investigators focused on age, duration of symptoms, preoperative symptom severity, neurophysiologic studies, type of transposition, and workers' compensation status but failed to find predictive factors affecting outcomes. Novak and colleagues[39] suggested that smoking might play a role in outcome after submuscular transposition and found that greater improvement was reported among nonsmokers than smokers at 2 years (level IV).

Traditionally, subluxation has been thought to be an indication for anterior transposition, but the determination of subluxation is largely subjective and there is not a uniform consensus. Calfee and colleagues[40] evaluated patients for ulnar nerve subluxation and found 37% of asymptomatic volunteers demonstrated nerve hypermobility.

Keith and Wollstein[41] performed submuscular transposition after making an intraoperative determination of instability and found that preoperative clinical examination was not a reliable predictor of intraoperative instability (level 4), noting a 14% rate of subluxation, which is lower than reported by Bartels and colleagues[42] (27%) (level I), who demonstrated outcome was not related to the presence of intraoperative subluxation by documenting the stability of the nerve without changing the surgical treatment and noting no difference in outcomes between those with and without with intraoperative subluxation.

Endoscopic Decompression

Thorough reviews of the surgical technique for endoscopic decompression of the ulnar nerve have been published previously.[43,44] Outcomes have reported 70% to 94% good to excellent results at 6 months to 4 years, suggesting results similar to other techniques are reproducible using endoscopic or minimally invasive techniques.[44–47] Reported complications include 30% rate of postoperative hematoma and a 12% rate of transient hypoesthesias in the MABC nerve distribution that resolved at 3 months. Intraoperative subluxation of the nerve requiring conversion to an open medial epicondylectomy was described in 6 of 21 procedures.[48] Comparison of open and endoscopic techniques was reported by Watts and Bain who prospectively collected patient-reported outcomes and reported equivalent results between cohorts at 12 months, with a trend toward improved satisfaction in the endoscopic group[49] (level III). The open cohort had more complications (40% vs 11%), including scar tenderness and mild numbness around the medial elbow.

Revision Surgery

Similar to other procedures involving ulnar nerve surgery, the literature on this topic is limited to retrospective case series and descriptions of techniques. Persistent symptoms may exist and are reported in up to 35% of procedures.[2] Goldfarb and colleagues[50] reported a 7% failure rate after primary in situ decompression at 4-year follow-up (level IV) and similar rates of 8% to 10% have been reported for submuscular anterior transposition and partial medial epicondylectomy.[51,52] Pathology identified at the revision procedure includes nerve compression at a remote site from the index surgery, inadequate decompression, cicatrix or scar formation, neuromas, and nerve subluxation. Submuscular transposition is commonly performed for revision surgery.[1] Vogel and coworkers[53] reported 55% good to excellent

outcomes at 3 years after revision to submuscular position for failed subcutaneous anterior transposition (level IV). Dagregorio and Saint-Cast[54] performed simple anterior neurolysis to treat failure after submuscular transposition and noted 90% good to excellent results, with 50% resolution on neurophysiologic testing (level IV). Autologous vein wrapping using the greater saphenous vein has been reported to improve visual analogue pain and function scores[55] (level IV). In cases of extensive scar formation, allograft biomatrix scaffolds (ie, GraftJacket, Wright Medical Technology, Arlington, TN, USA) have been used to wrap the nerve in a fashion similar to autologous vein wrapping but without the donor site morbidity from vein harvest[56] (level IV). Although anterior submuscular transposition is traditionally used as the revision procedure for failed surgery, the literature does not demonstrate one procedure is superior to another in terms of symptom relief or objective improvement.

COMPARATIVE LITERATURE
Nonrandomized Studies

Several nonrandomized, retrospective cohort studies comparing outcomes between in situ decompression, minimal and partial medial epicondylectomy, and anterior transposition to subcutaneous, submuscular, or intramuscular positions have not demonstrated differences in outcomes.[57–61] Keiner and colleagues[62] prospectively followed 33 patients for a minimum of 3 years and compared submuscular transposition with in situ decompression and found no differences in complication rates or outcomes, leading the investigators to recommend in situ decompression based on the thought that it is less invasive (level II). Mandelli and Baiguini[63] performed a prospective cohort study of patients with all McGowan grades; those with grade 1 underwent in situ decompression whereas those with grade 2/3 underwent either anterior transposition to a subcutaneous or submuscular position (level II). Patients undergoing in situ decompression demonstrated 84% excellent results compared with 33% and 8% for subcutaneous and submuscular transpositions, respectively. Interpretation of this result is difficult, however, given existing literature, suggesting poorer outcomes for patients with more severe stages of the Dellon classification.

Using a decision analysis model, Brauer and Graham[64] compared 4 procedures using complete relief of sensory symptoms for at least 2 years as the primary measure of a good outcome (level I). The analysis showed that for moderate-to-severe UNE symptoms, in situ decompression had the highest expected utility or the most desirable outcome while accounting for potential complications, with subcutaneous anterior transposition closely in second place. The investigators found that this result held until the complication rate for in situ decompression in the model was increased to 82% (an unrealistically high percentage). This argues for in situ decompression as the primary treatment for UNE and reserving epicondylectomy or transposition for those patients where revision surgery is required.

Randomized Studies

Prospective RCTs are not common for ulnar neuropathy because there is not even a consensus on diagnosis or treatment indications. Some surgeons rely on objective findings of electrodiagnostic (EDX) studies for diagnosis, whereas other surgeons think it is primarily clinical.[65] Some investigators advocate surgical treatment in patients with clinical symptoms and negative EDX studies,[66] whereas other investigators suggest that up to 50% of these patients show spontaneous clinical improvement with nonoperative management.[67] Variation in surgical techniques between investigators also makes comparative studies difficult to interpret.

Despite these limitations, several RCTs exist.[42,68–71] Bartels and colleagues[42] randomized patients with EDX evidence of UNE to either in situ decompression or subcutaneous anterior transposition (level I). At 1 year, there were no statistically significant differences in terms of the percentage of patients with good to excellent outcomes but a higher complication rate was noted in the transposition cohort, largely due to hypoesthesia in the region of the incision as well as a higher incidence of postoperative infection (9% vs 2%). Similar results were reported by Nabhan and colleagues,[70] who found no differences in outcome for in situ decompression compared with subcutaneous anterior transposition at 9 months and thus recommend in situ decompression (level I). In 2005, Gervasio and coworkers performed an RCT in 70 patients with severe (Dellon grade 3) neuropathy to evaluate in situ decompression and submuscular anterior transposition[69] (level I). No significant differences were noted in EDX or clinical outcome, which correlated with the existing literature for either method with 80% and 82% good to excellent outcomes reported for in situ decompression and submuscular anterior transposition, respectively. These investigators did not have any major complications in either group. Zarezadeh and colleagues[71] reported on 48 patients randomized to subcutaneous or submuscular

transposition and found more improvement in postoperative pain levels with submuscular transposition (level I).

Biggs and Curtis[68] randomized 44 patients to in situ decompression or submuscular anterior transposition and reported their 1-year outcomes, McGowan grade, and complication rates (level I). At final follow-up, there were no differences between the groups even when controlling for preoperative grade and examining only the most severe cases. Importantly, however, the submuscular transposition group had more complications, including 3 cases of deep wound infection requiring intravenous antibiotics and 2 cases of re-exploration. The investigators hypothesized that the increased dissection necessary to perform a submuscular transposition may have created increased potential space, which, along with an increased operative time for submuscular transposition, may explain the increased risk of infection among these patients. Therefore, these investigators also suggest in situ decompression be performed for primary UNE.

Meta-Analyses

Since the 1998 report by Bartels and colleagues,[17] 1 meta-analysis of level I studies[72] and 1 Cochrane review[73] have been published and together these studies represent the highest level of evidence to date on the management of UNE. Similar analyses have been performed previously[74,75]; however, these reports combined results from studies with lower levels of evidence and, therefore, represent a lower level of evidence themselves.[76] Both Zlodowski and colleagues[72] and Caliandro and colleagues[73] included the same 4 randomized studies in their analysis (discussed previously).[42,68–70] Although the investigators used different statistical pooling methods, both found similar conclusions. There was no difference in the risk ratio for clinical or neurophysiologic improvement between in situ decompression and anterior transposition and significantly more wound infections were found associated with transposition.[73] Based on this evidence, the investigators were unable to recommend one treatment as the best identifiable procedure for UNE and are further unable to identify when patients should be treated operatively or conservatively.

SUMMARY

On the basis of the authors' review of the literature, preoperative determination of which patients will benefit from which type of procedure is not possible at this time. In the authors' practice, simple decompression is performed, either by open or endoscopic techniques, for primary cases. An effort is made to determine if the nerve subluxes preoperatively, as described by Calfee and colleagues.[40] For perching nerves, the nerve is left in its native position and for nerves that sublux anterior to the epicondyle, a transposition in the subcutaneous plane is performed. Although subluxation is not an absolute indication to perform transposition, the literature demonstrates outcomes for revision surgery are not as good as primary surgery; thus, the nerve is transposed in hopes of decreasing the need for revision surgery. Submuscular transposition is reserved for revision cases or active patients with minimal subcutaneous tissue where the nerve is thought at risk for irritation in the subcutaneous position. The authors are aware of current studies to validate outcomes for treatment of UNE, which is the next step in determining the optimal treatment, but they are yet to be published.

REFERENCES

1. Elhassan B, Steinmann SP. Entrapment neuropathy of the ulnar nerve. J Am Acad Orthop Surg 2007; 15(11):672–81.

2. Gellman H. Compression of the ulnar nerve at the elbow: cubital tunnel syndrome. Instr Course Lect 2008;57:187–9.

3. Palmer BA, Hughes TB. Cubital tunnel syndrome. J Hand Surg Am 2010;35(1):153–6.

4. Green JR Jr, Rayan GM. The cubital tunnel: anatomic, histologic, and biomechanical study. J Shoulder Elbow Surg 1999;8(5):466–70.

5. Gelberman RH, Yamaguchi K, Hollstien SB, et al. Changes in interstitial pressure and cross-sectional area of the cubital tunnel and of the ulnar nerve with flexion of the elbow. An experimental study in human cadavera. J Bone Joint Surg Am 1998;80(4):492–501.

6. Wright TW, Glowczewskie F Jr, Cowin D, et al. Ulnar nerve excursion and strain at the elbow and wrist associated with upper extremity motion. J Hand Surg Am 2001;26(4):655–62.

7. Siemionow M, Agaoglu G, Hoffmann R. Anatomic characteristics of a fascia and its bands overlying the ulnar nerve in the proximal forearm: a cadaver study. J Hand Surg Eur Vol 2007;32(3): 302–7.

8. Kleinman WB. Cubital tunnel syndrome: anterior transposition as a logical approach to complete nerve decompression. J Hand Surg Am 1999; 24(5):886–97.

9. Heithoff SJ. Cubital tunnel syndrome does not require transposition of the ulnar nerve. J Hand Surg Am 1999;24(5):898–905.

10. McGowan AJ. The results of transposition of the ulnar nerve for traumatic ulnar neuritis. J Bone Joint Surg Br 1950;32(3):293–301.

11. Goldberg BJ, Light TR, Blair SJ. Ulnar neuropathy at the elbow: results of medial epicondylectomy. J Hand Surg Am 1989;14(2 Pt 1):182–8.

12. Dellon AL. Review of treatment results for ulnar nerve entrapment at the elbow. J Hand Surg Am 1989;14(4):688–700.

13. Levine DW, Simmons BP, Koris MJ, et al. A self-administered questionnaire for the assessment of severity of symptoms and functional status in carpal tunnel syndrome. J Bone Joint Surg Am 1993;75(11):1585–92.

14. Wilson DH, Krout R. Surgery of ulnar neuropathy at the elbow: 16 cases treated by decompression without transposition. Technical note. J Neurosurg 1973;38(6):780–5.

15. Macadam SA, Bezuhly M, Lefaivre KA. Outcomes measures used to assess results after surgery for cubital tunnel syndrome: a systematic review of the literature. J Hand Surg Am 2009;34(8): 1482–91.e5.

16. Mondelli M, Padua L, Giannini F, et al. A self-administered questionnaire of ulnar neuropathy at the elbow. Neurol Sci 2006;27(6):402–11.

17. Bartels RH, Menovsky T, Van Overbeeke JJ, et al. Surgical management of ulnar nerve compression at the elbow: an analysis of the literature. J Neurosurg 1998;89(5):722–7.

18. Karthik K, Nanda R, Storey S, et al. Severe ulnar nerve entrapment at the elbow: functional outcome after minimally invasive in situ decompression. J Hand Surg 2012;37(2):115–22.

19. Pavelka M, Rhomberg M, Estermann D, et al. Decompression without anterior transposition: an effective minimally invasive technique for cubital tunnel syndrome. Minim Invasive Neurosurg 2004; 47(2):119–23.

20. Nathan PA, Istvan JA, Meadows KD. Intermediate and long-term outcomes following simple decompression of the ulnar nerve at the elbow. Chir Main 2005;24(1):29–34.

21. Taniguchi Y, Takami M, Takami T, et al. Simple decompression with small skin incision for cubital tunnel syndrome. J Hand Surg Br 2002;27(6):559–62.

22. Amako M, Nemoto K, Kawaguchi M, et al. Comparison between partial and minimal medial epicondylectomy combined with decompression for the treatment of cubital tunnel syndrome. J Hand Surg Am 2000;25(6):1043–50.

23. Efstathopoulos DG, Themistocleous GS, Papagelopoulos PJ, et al. Outcome of partial medial epicondylectomy for cubital tunnel syndrome. Clin Orthop Relat Res 2006;444:134–9.

24. Kim KW, Lee HJ, Rhee SH, et al. Minimal epicondylectomy improves neurologic deficits in moderate

to severe cubital tunnel syndrome. Clin Orthop Relat Res 2012;470(5):1405–13.

25. Muermans S, De Smet L. Partial medial epicondylectomy for cubital tunnel syndrome: outcome and complications. J Shoulder Elbow Surg 2002; 11(3):248–52.

26. Seradge H, Owen W. Cubital tunnel release with medial epicondylectomy factors influencing the outcome. J Hand Surg Am 1998;23(3):483–91.

27. Kleinman WB, Bishop AT. Anterior intramuscular transposition of the ulnar nerve. J Hand Surg Am 1989;14(6):972–9.

28. Hashiguchi H, Ito H, Sawaizumi T. Stabilized subcutaneous transposition of the ulnar nerve. Int Orthop 2003;27(4):232–4.

29. Gokay NS, Bagatur AE. Subcutaneous anterior transposition of the ulnar nerve in cubital tunnel syndrome. Acta Orthop Traumatol Turc 2012; 46(4):243–9.

30. Lascar T, Laulan J. Cubital tunnel syndrome: a retrospective review of 53 anterior subcutaneous transpositions. J Hand Surg Br 2000;25(5):453–6.

31. Hamidreza A, Saeid A, Mohammadreza D, et al. Anterior subcutaneous transposition of ulnar nerve with fascial flap and complete excision of medial intermuscular septum in cubital tunnel syndrome: a prospective patient cohort. Clin Neurol Neurosurg 2011;113(8):631–4.

32. Iba K, Wada T, Tamakawa M, et al. Diffusion-weighted magnetic resonance imaging of the ulnar nerve in cubital tunnel syndrome. Hand Surg 2010; 15(1):11–5.

33. Davis GA, Bulluss KJ. Submuscular transposition of the ulnar nerve: review of safety, efficacy and correlation with neurophysiological outcome. J Clin Neurosci 2005;12(5):524–8.

34. Fitzgerald BT, Dao KD, Shin AY. Functional outcomes in young, active duty, military personnel after submuscular ulnar nerve transposition. J Hand Surg Am 2004;29(4):619–24.

35. Pell RF 4th, Velyvis JH, Chahal R, et al. Functional outcome following anterior submuscular transposition of the ulnar nerve with V-Y lengthening of the flexor-pronator origin. Am J Orthop (Belle Mead NJ) 2004;33(6):290–4.

36. Charles YP, Coulet B, Rouzaud JC, et al. Comparative clinical outcomes of submuscular and subcutaneous transposition of the ulnar nerve for cubital tunnel syndrome. J Hand Surg Am 2009; 34(5):866–74.

37. Kose KC, Bilgin S, Cebesoy O, et al. Clinical results versus subjective improvement with anterior transposition in cubital tunnel syndrome. Adv Ther 2007; 24(5):996–1005.

38. Shi Q, MacDermid JC, Santaguida PL, et al. Predictors of surgical outcomes following anterior transposition of ulnar nerve for cubital tunnel syndrome: a systematic review. J Hand Surg Am 2011;36(12):1996–2001.e1–6.

39. Novak CB, Mackinnon SE, Stuebe AM. Patient self-reported outcome after ulnar nerve transposition. Ann Plast Surg 2002;48(3):274–80.

40. Calfee RP, Manske PR, Gelberman RH, et al. Clinical assessment of the ulnar nerve at the elbow: reliability of instability testing and the association of hypermobility with clinical symptoms. J Bone Joint Surg Am 2010;92(17):2801–8.

41. Keith J, Wollstein R. A tailored approach to the surgical treatment of cubital tunnel syndrome. Ann Plast Surg 2011;66(6):637–9.

42. Bartels RH, Verhagen WI, van der Wilt GJ, et al. Prospective randomized controlled study comparing simple decompression versus anterior subcutaneous transposition for idiopathic neuropathy of the ulnar nerve at the elbow: part 1. Neurosurgery 2005;56(3):522–30 [discussion: 522–30].

43. Cobb TK. Endoscopic cubital tunnel release. J Hand Surg Am 2010;35(10):1690–7.

44. Hoffmann R, Siemionow M. The endoscopic management of cubital tunnel syndrome. J Hand Surg Br 2006;31(1):23–9.

45. Flores LP. Endoscopically assisted release of the ulnar nerve for cubital tunnel syndrome. Acta Neurochir 2010;152(4):619–25.

46. Tsai TM, Chen IC, Majd ME, et al. Cubital tunnel release with endoscopic assistance: results of a new technique. J Hand Surg Am 1999;24(1):21–9.

47. Yoshida A, Okutsu I, Hamanaka I. Endoscopic anatomical nerve observation and minimally invasive management of cubital tunnel syndrome. J Hand Surg 2009;34(1):115–20.

48. Ward WA, Siffri PC. Endoscopically assisted ulnar neurolysis for cubital tunnel syndrome. Tech Hand Up Extrem Surg 2009;13(3):155–9.

49. Watts AC, Bain GI. Patient-rated outcome of ulnar nerve decompression: a comparison of endoscopic and open in situ decompression. J Hand Surg Am 2009;34(8):1492–8.

50. Goldfarb CA, Sutter MM, Martens EJ, et al. Incidence of re-operation and subjective outcome following in situ decompression of the ulnar nerve at the cubital tunnel. J Hand Surg 2009;34(3): 379–83.

51. Schnabl SM, Kisslinger F, Schramm A, et al. Subjective outcome, neurophysiological investigations, postoperative complications and recurrence rate of partial medial epicondylectomy in cubital tunnel syndrome. Arch Orthop Trauma Surg 2011; 131(8):1027–33.

52. Dellon AL, Coert JH. Results of the musculofascial lengthening technique for submuscular transposition of the ulnar nerve at the elbow. J Bone Joint Surg Am 2004;86(Suppl 1(Pt 2)): 169–79.

53. Vogel RB, Nossaman BC, Rayan GM. Revision anterior submuscular transposition of the ulnar nerve for failed subcutaneous transposition. Br J Plast Surg 2004;57(4):311–6.

54. Dagregorio G, Saint-Cast Y. Simple neurolysis for failed anterior submuscular transposition of the ulnar nerve at the elbow. Int Orthop 2004;28(6):342–6.

55. Kokkalis ZT, Jain S, Sotereanos DG. Vein wrapping at cubital tunnel for ulnar nerve problems. J Shoulder Elbow Surg 2010;19(Suppl 2):91–7.

56. Puckett BN, Gaston RG, Lourie GM. A novel technique for the treatment of recurrent cubital tunnel syndrome: ulnar nerve wrapping with a tissue engineered bioscaffold. J Hand Surg 2011;36(2):130–4.

57. Taha A, Galarza M, Zuccarello M, et al. Outcomes of cubital tunnel surgery among patients with absent sensory nerve conduction. Neurosurgery 2004;54(4):891–5.

58. Hahn SB, Choi YR, Kang HJ, et al. Decompression of the ulnar nerve and minimal medial epicondylectomy with a small incision for cubital tunnel syndrome: comparison with anterior subcutaneous transposition of the nerve. J Plast Reconstr Aesthet Surg 2010;63(7):1150–5.

59. Baek GH, Kwon BC, Chung MS. Comparative study between minimal medial epicondylectomy and anterior subcutaneous transposition of the ulnar nerve for cubital tunnel syndrome. J Shoulder Elbow Surg 2006;15(5):609–13.

60. Matsuzaki H, Yoshizu T, Maki Y, et al. Long-term clinical and neurologic recovery in the hand after surgery for severe cubital tunnel syndrome. J Hand Surg Am 2004;29(3):373–8.

61. Asamoto S, Boker DK, Jodicke A. Surgical treatment for ulnar nerve entrapment at the elbow. Neurol Med 2005;45(5):240–4.

62. Keiner D, Gaab MR, Schroeder HW, et al. Comparison of the long-term results of anterior transposition of the ulnar nerve or simple decompression in the treatment of cubital tunnel syndrome–a prospective study. Acta Neurochir 2009;151(4):311–5.

63. Mandelli C, Baiguini M. Ulnar nerve entrapment neuropathy at the elbow: decisional algorithm and surgical considerations. Neurocirugia (Astur) 2009;20(1):31–8.

64. Brauer CA, Graham B. The surgical treatment of cubital tunnel syndrome: a decision analysis. J Hand Surg 2007;32(6):654–62.

65. Hutchison RL, Rayan G. Diagnosis of cubital tunnel syndrome. J Hand Surg Am 2011;36(9):1519–21.

66. Tomaino MM, Brach PJ, Vansickle DP. The rationale for and efficacy of surgical intervention for electrodiagnostic-negative cubital tunnel syndrome. J Hand Surg Am 2001;26(6):1077–81.

67. Padua L, Aprile I, Caliandro P, et al. Natural history of ulnar entrapment at elbow. Clin Neurophysiol 2002;113(12):1980–4.

68. Biggs M, Curtis JA. Randomized, prospective study comparing ulnar neurolysis in situ with submuscular transposition. Neurosurgery 2006;58(2):296–304 [discussion: 296–304].

69. Gervasio O, Gambardella G, Zaccone C, et al. Simple decompression versus anterior submuscular transposition of the ulnar nerve in severe cubital tunnel syndrome: a prospective randomized study. Neurosurgery 2005;56(1):108–17.

70. Nabhan A, Ahlhelm F, Kelm J, et al. Simple decompression or subcutaneous anterior transposition of the ulnar nerve for cubital tunnel syndrome. J Hand Surg Br 2005;30(5):521–4.

71. Zarezadeh A, Semshaki H, Nourbakhsh M. Comparison of anterior subcutaneous and submuscular transposition of ulnar nerve in treatment of cubital tunnel syndrome: a prospective randomized trial. J Res Med Sci 2012;17:745–9.

72. Zlowodzki M, Chan S, Bhandari M, et al. Anterior transposition compared with simple decompression for treatment of cubital tunnel syndrome. A meta-analysis of randomized, controlled trials. J Bone Joint Surg Am 2007;89(12):2591–8.

73. Caliandro P, La Torre G, Padua R, et al. Treatment for ulnar neuropathy at the elbow. Cochrane Database Syst Rev 2012;(7):CD006839.

74. Mowlavi A, Andrews K, Lille S, et al. The management of cubital tunnel syndrome: a meta-analysis of clinical studies. Plast Reconstr Surg 2000;106(2):327–34.

75. Macadam SA, Gandhi R, Bezuhly M, et al. Simple decompression versus anterior subcutaneous and submuscular transposition of the ulnar nerve for cubital tunnel syndrome: a meta-analysis. J Hand Surg Am 2008;33(8):1314.e1–12.

76. Wright RW, Brand RA, Dunn W, et al. How to write a systematic review. Clin Orthop Relat Res 2007;455:23–9.

Uncommon Upper Extremity Compression Neuropathies

Elisa J. Knutsen, MD, Ryan P. Calfee, MD, MSc*

KEYWORDS

- Compression • Median • Nerve • Radial • Ulnar • Uncommon

KEY POINTS

- Radial tunnel syndrome often accompanies lateral epicondylitis but is best distinguished on physical examination by the location of tenderness over the mobile wad as opposed to the extensor carpi radialis brevis.
- Compression of the motor branch of the ulnar nerve in Guyon's canal should be suspected in patients with demonstrable intrinsic muscle weakness (hypothenar's, interossei, adductor pollicis) without sensory disturbance.
- Pronator syndrome may be suspected in patients with a history consistent with carpal tunnel syndrome without demonstrable provocative signs at the carpal tunnel.
- Spontaneous anterior interosseous nerve palsy is typically treated nonoperatively with expected recovery within 1 year.

INTRODUCTION

Carpal tunnel syndrome is the most common compression neuropathy in the upper extremity. The annual incidence of carpal tunnel syndrome is between 0.1% and 0.35% compared with a 0.02% annual incidence of ulnar nerve compression syndromes or a 0.003% annual incidence of radial nerve compression syndromes.[1,2] Although rare, it is important to recognize uncommon nerve compression syndromes. This article reviews the uncommon compression syndromes/palsies of the radial, ulnar, and median nerves. These conditions are uncommon. Most publications are small retrospective series or case reports, so treatment decisions are not typically based on high levels of evidence; but given the rarity of these conditions, this will likely not change in the near future.

RADIAL NERVE
Anatomy

The radial nerve is the terminal branch of the posterior cord of the brachial plexus. Posterior to the axillary artery, the nerve travels through the triangular interval and then continues along the spiral groove of the humerus. Approximately 11 cm proximal to the elbow, the nerve is in the posterior compartment and penetrates the lateral intermuscular septum to enter the anterior compartment of the arm.[3] It continues distally and enters the forearm anterior to the lateral epicondyle where it divides into the superficial and deep branches approximately 3 to 4 cm proximal to the leading edge of the supinator.[4] The deep branch, the posterior interosseous nerve (PIN), passes beneath the supinator as shown in **Fig. 1**. The superficial branch of the radial nerve (SBRN) travels distally

Disclosures: None.
Department of Orthopaedic Surgery, Washington University School of Medicine, Washington University, 660 South Euclid Avenue, Campus Box 8233, St Louis, MO 63110, USA
* Corresponding author.
E-mail address: calfee@wudosis.wustl.edu

Hand Clin 29 (2013) 443–453
http://dx.doi.org/10.1016/j.hcl.2013.04.014
0749-0712/13/$ – see front matter © 2013 Elsevier Inc. All rights reserved.

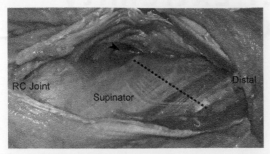

Fig. 1. View from lateral elbow between ECRB (extensor carpi radialis brevis) and EDC (extensor digitorum communis) origins with PIN (*arrowhead*) entering and coursing under supinator (*dotted path*). RC, radiocapitellar.

on the undersurface of the brachioradialis, becoming subcutaneous in the distal one-third of the forearm where it pierces between the brachioradialis and extensor carpi radialis longus (ECRL) tendons to provide sensation to the dorsoradial aspect of the hand.[5] Depending on the point of compression, patients may suffer from 3 distinct radial nerve compression syndromes: radial tunnel syndrome, posterior interosseous syndrome, and superficial radial nerve compression (Wartenberg syndrome).

RADIAL TUNNEL SYNDROME

In 1972, Roles and Maudsley[6] introduced radial tunnel syndrome (RTS) as a refractory lateral epicondylitis caused by compression of the PIN within the radial tunnel and advocated surgically decompressing the radial nerve. RTS is now understood to present with pain in the proximal lateral forearm with tenderness to palpation 4 to 6 cm distal to the lateral epicondyle. Often the pain is worse with repetitive supination and pronation. RTS is distinguished from posterior interosseous syndrome by a lack of motor weakness.

The radial tunnel begins anterior to the radiocapitellar joint and is approximately 5 cm in length. It extends from the lateral epicondyle of humerus to the distal edge of the supinator muscle, bounded by the brachioradialis and extensor carpi radialis longus laterally and the brachialis and biceps brachii tendon medially. The floor of the tunnel is the anterior capsule of the radiocapitellar joint and the deep layer of supinator muscle. The extensor carpi radialis brevis and the superficial layer of the supinator muscle form the roof.

RTS is the result of compression of the nerve by one of the following structures: the superficial layer of the supinator muscle (arcade of Frohse), the tendinous margins of the extensor carpi radialis brevis, the leash of Henry (vessels from the radial

recurrent artery), or fibrous bands distal to the radial head.[7] In a cadaveric study of 46 upper limbs, Konjengbam and Elangbam[8] found that in 87% of specimens, the superficial layer of the supinator muscle was tendinous, which is considered the most common cause of RTS.

Diagnosis

RTS is based solely on clinical evaluation because neither advanced imaging nor electrodiagnostic studies demonstrate an objective source or location of nerve compression and no pathognomonic diagnostic finding exists.[9,10] Generally, tenderness to palpation along the proximal radial forearm in the supinator muscle and 4 to 6 cm distal to the lateral epicondyle that simulates the patients' pain is considered most suggestive of this diagnosis.[6] The classic clinical test for RTS is pain with resisted supination while the shoulder is adducted and the elbow is flexed to 90°. Pain with resisted middle finger extension has also been proposed as a diagnostic examination maneuver.[11] Some investigators consider relief with an anesthetic injection at the point of maximal tenderness to be diagnostic of RTS if the injection also produces transient radial nerve palsy.[12,13]

The diagnosis of RTS can be complicated by other conditions that cause pain in the area, such as lateral epicondylitis or lower cervical radiculopathy.[14] The incidence of coexisting lateral epicondylitis has been reported to be as high as 43%.[13,15]

Treatment

The initial treatment of RTS is nonoperative and includes rest, antiinflammatory medication, and activity modification to avoid activities that require elbow extension, forearm pronation, and wrist extension. If that fails, a steroid injection at the point of maximal tenderness may provide relief. In one study, 16 out of 25 patients with RTS had relief that lasted 2 years following an injection of 40 mg of triamcinolone.[12] If symptoms persist, surgical options can be considered; however, *there are no natural history or randomized trials comparing nonsurgical versus surgical interventions.*[16]

Retrospective outcomes following radial nerve decompression are varied, with success rates from 10% to 95% as shown in **Table 1**. In most of these studies, success is defined as having an excellent or good outcome according to the Roles and Maudsley criteria. According to these criteria, an excellent outcome is defined as complete resolution of pain and the return of full range of motion and activity. A good outcome is defined as occasional discomfort but with full range of motion.[6]

Table 1 Reported success rates of surgical interventions for RTS			
Author	Nerve Released	N	Success Rate n (%)
Roles & Maudsley,[6] 1972	SBRN/PIN	38	35 (92)
Hagert et al,[11] 1977	PIN	50	42 (84)
Lister et al,[7] 1979	PIN	20	19 (95)
Moss & Switzer,[14] 1983	PIN	15	14 (93)
Ritts et al,[15] 1987	PIN	39	29 (74)
Verhaar & Spaans,[9] 1991	PIN	10	1 (10)
Younge & Moise,[64] 1993	PIN	35	28 (80)
Atroshi et al,[21] 1995	PIN	37	13 (35)
Lawrence et al,[20] 1995	SRBN/PIN	30	21 (70)
Jebson & Engber,[65] 1997	SBRN/PIN	24	16 (67)
Sarhadi et al,[12] 1998	PIN	9	7 (78)
De Smet et al,[17] 1999	PIN	20	15 (75)
Sotereanos et al,[13] 1999	PIN	28	11 (39)
Lee et al,[18] 2008	PIN	27	22 (82)
Bolster & Bakker,[19] 2009	SBRN	12	11 (92)

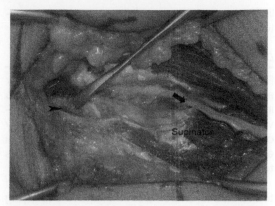

Fig. 2. View from lateral elbow after debriding lateral epicondyle (*arrowhead*) and decompressing the PIN (*arrow*) through the supinator (superficial head reflected).

Comparing the results of studies listed in **Table 1** is challenging because of the variation in diagnostic criteria, patient population, exact surgical treatment, and length of follow-up. Several of these studies combined patients who underwent isolated radial tunnel release with those who also had concomitant surgery, such as lateral epicondyle debridement or other nerve decompression surgeries.[13,17,18] **Fig. 2** shows an example of radial tunnel decompression performed concomitantly with debridement of the lateral epicondyle.

Most of the investigators listed in **Table 1** advocated for releasing the PIN at the radial tunnel for the treatment of RTS. However, Bolster and Bakker[19] suggested that the key to the success of the treatment is the release of the SBRN, and they report successful outcomes in 11 out of 12 patients that had only the SBRN released.[19]

Some of these studies also reported patient satisfaction.[20,21] According to De Smet,[17] satisfaction was higher among patients who had a combined lateral epicondylar muscle release radial tunnel decompression,[17] whereas Lee and colleagues[18] reported lower surgical success rates in patients with concomitant lateral epicondylitis or nerve compression syndromes. Patients who are being treated under workers' compensation or involved in litigation have poorer outcomes following surgery.[13]

Complications

The risks associated with decompressing the radial tunnel include partial or transient PIN palsy. Atroshi and colleagues[21] reported 2 cases of partial radial nerve paresis and 3 cases with diminished sensation in the radial nerve distribution following surgical release of the radial tunnel in 37 patients. In a study of 30 patients, Lawrence and colleagues[20] reported 1 case of transient PIN palsy, 3 cases of mild chronic regional pain syndrome, and 2 patients who had hyperesthesia in SRN distribution. Sotereanos and colleagues[13] reported that 11 out of 28 cases of radial tunnel release had temporary SRN neurapraxia and 1 patient had transient PIN palsy. In a series of 27 patients, Lee and colleagues[18] reported that 3 patients had a transient SBRN irritation that resolved within 12 months.

POSTERIOR INTEROSSEOUS NERVE SYNDROME

Posterior interosseous nerve syndrome (PINS) is a compression neuropathy of the PIN in the radial tunnel; however, unlike RTS, patients with PINS have a loss of motor function and do not have pain. Similar to RTS, compression of the PIN can be caused by fibrous bands within the radial tunnel or from mass effect from a benign tumor (eg, lipoma or ganglia) or synovitis related to rheumatoid arthritis.[22,23]

Diagnosis

Patients typically present with weakness in finger and thumb extension, but wrist extension remains intact because the extensor carpi radialis is innervated proximal to site of compression. PIN palsy can mimic extensor tendon ruptures, but clinical examination can differentiate by using tenodesis to evaluate the integrity of the extensor tendons.

Magnetic resonance imaging (MRI) can be used to evaluate for a lipoma or other space-occupying lesion that may be compressing the PIN. Electrodiagnostic studies can be used for confirmation of the clinical diagnosis and to quantify the severity of the muscular denervation.

Treatment

Like RTS, the initial treatment of PINS is nonoperative and includes rest, antiinflammatory medications, and activity modification. However, in the setting a PIN paralysis, surgery is indicated at 3 months if there is no sign of spontaneous recovery or sooner if a space-occupying lesion is identified.

Because the same nerve is being compressed in both RTS and PINS, the surgical approach is similar. The radial tunnel is explored and decompressed, and any compressing lesions are also addressed. In their report of nontraumatic paralysis of the PIN, Hashizume and colleagues[24] reported that PIN paralysis recovered in 24 of the 25 patients treated surgically between 2 and 18 months (mean 5.6 months). In a smaller study, Vrieling and colleagues[25] reported good to excellent results in 5 of the 8 patients treated with nerve decompression.

WARTENBERG SYNDROME

Wartenberg syndrome is compression of the SBRN. Approximately 9 cm proximal to the radial styloid, the SBRN becomes subcutaneous traveling distally between the brachioradialis and the ECRL tendons. The nerve can be compressed anywhere along its course but is at greatest risk during this transition from a deep to subcutaneous structure. External trauma, such as from a tight watchband or handcuffs, is a common cause of SBRN irritation distally near the radial styloid.[26]

Patients with Wartenberg syndrome typically present with paresthesias along the dorsal radial forearm radiating to the thumb, index, and long fingers. If patients also have weakness in the PIN innervated muscles, a more proximal lesion or diagnosis involving the cervical spine or proper radial nerve should be considered. A positive Tinel sign over the course of the SBRN is the most common physical finding. However, patients may also have pain with ulnar deviation similar to de Quervain tenosynovitis, and nerve irritability may coexist with inflammation within the first dorsal extensor compartment.

Spontaneous resolution of Wartenberg syndrome is common. Therefore, treatment should focus on nonoperative measures, such as the removal of external compression, splinting, rest, and nonsteroidal antiinflammatory medications. In their study of 50 patients with Wartenberg syndrome, Lanzetta and Foucher[27] reported an excellent or good outcome in 71% of the 29 patients with nonoperative management, which included the removal of a tight watch strap, splinting, or a corticosteroid injection. In their series, 50% of their patients were also diagnosed with de Quervain tenosynovitis. They offered surgical decompression to patients who failed nonoperative treatment and reported a 74% success rate in those 23 patients. The success rate for surgery on the superficial radial nerve at the level of the radial styloid is modest as Calfee and colleagues[28] noted that 11 of 20 patients continued to report neurogenic symptoms 3.5 years after neurolysis.

Authors' Experience

In the authors' practice, most patients with RTS have presented with concomitant lateral epicondylitis, which has often followed the use of a forearm strap. Discontinuation of the forearm strap and pursuing alternative forms of treatment of the lateral epicondylitis generally results in resolution of the radial tunnel symptoms. Because radial tunnel is purely a subjective diagnosis, the authors are hesitant to offer surgical treatment. Similarly in the distal forearm, the authors seek to identify what are often external causes of superficial radial nerve irritation. Treatment should be directed at decreasing pain, and the authors think that residual nonpainful paresthesia is not an indication for surgery given the possibility of inciting more painful neurologic symptoms.

ULNAR TUNNEL SYNDROME

Ulnar tunnel syndrome is defined as a compressive neuropathy of the ulnar nerve at the wrist. Dupont and colleagues[29] first used the term *ulnar tunnel syndrome* in 1965 to describe 4 of their patients with ulnar neuritis from various causes. The ulnar tunnel is an obliquely oriented fibroosseous tunnel located at the level of the carpus that contains the ulnar nerve, ulnar artery, and communicating veins and fat. The ulnar tunnel is often referred to as the Guyon canal, but Guyon actually described a space at the base of the hypothenar eminence where the ulnar nerve bifurcates and is vulnerable to compression.[30] There are numerous reported causes for compression of the ulnar nerve within the ulnar tunnel. Compression can occur because of space-occupying masses, such as ganglion cysts; repetitive trauma; edema from local trauma, such as metacarpal or carpal fractures; or from a vascular lesion, such as thromboangiitis of the ulnar vessels.[31,32]

Typically, compression of the ulnar nerve at the wrist is categorized into 3 types depending on the clinical deficits: sensory, motor, or mixed symptoms.[31] In their cadaveric study of the ulnar tunnel, Gross and Gelberman[30] described the 3 zones of the tunnel that correlate to the clinical picture (**Fig. 3**). Zone 1 is the portion of the tunnel proximal to the ulnar nerve bifurcation where the nerve contains 2 groups of distinct fascicles: the palmar-radial fibers that become the superficial sensory branch of the ulnar nerve and the dorsal ulnar fibers that become the deep motor branch. Zone 2 encompasses the deep motor branch of the nerve, and zone 3 surrounds the superficial sensory branch of the ulnar nerve. Lesions arising from the deep surface of the ulnar tunnel should compress motor fibers first because the motor fascicles are located posteriorly throughout zone 1. Similarly, superficial lesions or compression in this zone should affect the sensory fascicles and cause sensory symptoms first.[30]

Anatomy

The ulnar nerve originates from the medial cord (C8-T1) of the brachial plexus and courses through the axilla into the anterior compartment of the arm. It then pierces the intermuscular septum to enter the posterior compartment and travels posterior to the medial epicondyle through the cubital tunnel. The nerve enters the forearm between the 2 heads of the flexor carpi ulnaris and continues distally on the surface of the flexor digitorum profundus. The dorsal cutaneous nerve separates from the main nerve 6 cm proximal to the ulnar styloid and becomes subcutaneous 5.0 cm proximal to the pisiform.[33] This nerve provides sensation to the dorsal ulnar aspect of the hand and the small and ulnar aspect of the ring finger.

The ulnar nerve proper then travels superficially to enter the ulnar tunnel. The entrance to the tunnel is triangular in cross section and begins at the volar carpal ligament, which is approximately 2.5 mm proximal to the pisiform. The ulnar tunnel is 40 to 45 mm in length with the wrist in neutral and ends at the fibrous arch of the hypothenar muscles.[30,34] The anatomic boundaries of the canal vary along its length. From proximal to distal, the medial border is the flexor carpi ulnaris tendon sheath, the pisiform, and the abductor digiti minimi. Laterally, the flexor tendons, the transverse carpal ligament, and the hook of the hamate define the tunnel. The roof of the canal is the volar carpal ligament, palmaris brevis, and the hypothenar connective tissue. The floor of the canal consists of the transverse carpal, the pisohamate and the pisometacarpal ligaments, and the opponens digiti minimi muscle.[30]

The contents of the canal include the ulnar nerve, ulnar artery, veins, and fatty tissue. The nerve is deep and ulnar to the ulnar artery. Within the canal, the nerve bifurcates into the superficial sensory and deep motor branches about 6 mm distal to the distal edge of the pisiform.[34] The superficial branch supplies the palmaris brevis and provides sensibility to the ulnar hypothenar eminence, the small finger, and ulnar half of the ring finer. The deep motor branch gives off a branch that supplies the hypothenar muscles and travels deep and radially between abductor digiti minimi and flexor digiti minimi. As it crosses the palm, it innervates the dorsal interossei, the third and fourth lumbricals, the adductor pollicis, and the flexor pollicis brevis and terminates in the first dorsal interossei.

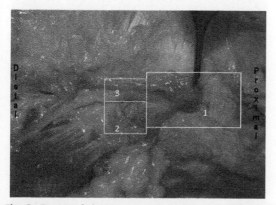

Fig. 3. Zones of the Guyon canal: zone 1 over mixed ulnar nerve, zone 2 encompassing motor branch ulnar nerve, zone 3 of sensory branches after exit of motor branch.

Cause

Multiple causes have been identified for ulnar tunnel syndrome. Ganglion cysts followed by fractures are the most common causes of ulnar nerve compression at the wrist.[35] Causes of ulnar nerve compression at the ulnar tunnel include ulnar artery thrombosis or aneurysm, anomalous muscles that cause ulnar nerve compression, and intraneural ganglions.[32,36,37] Prolonged bicycling has also been identified as causing distal ulnar nerve compression, known as cyclist's palsy, from leaning on the handlebars and direct pressure on the wrist.[38,39]

Ulnar tunnel syndrome is associated with and potentially caused by carpal tunnel syndrome.[40] Ablove and colleagues[41] demonstrated that both open or endoscopic carpal tunnel release reduces the pressure within the carpal and ulnar tunnels, which may support performing only a carpal tunnel release in patients with median and ulnar nerve compression at the wrist.

Diagnosis

The diagnosis of ulnar nerve compression at the wrist can be overlooked because most patients with neurologic symptoms on the ulnar hand have cubital tunnel syndrome or symptoms originating from the cervical spine. Patients with ulnar tunnel syndrome can present with purely motor or sensory symptoms or a combination of symptoms. They may report ulnar-sided wrist pain, weakness with pinch or grip, lack of coordination, or numbness or tingling in the small and ring fingers. Ulnar tunnel syndrome should not produce paresthesia on the dorsal-ulnar hand because the dorsal cutaneous ulnar nerve branches from the ulnar nerve proximal to the ulnar tunnel. Practitioners should elicit a history of repetitive trauma to the hypothenar region, prolonged bicycle riding, or recent trauma to the hand.

Physical Examination

The physical examination should include a complete neuromuscular examination and, in particular, an inspection for hypothenar atrophy, 2-point discrimination, and an Allen test to check the competency of the ulnar artery. Point tenderness over the hook of the hamate may indicate a fracture that could contribute to ulnar nerve compression. In a study of 31 patients with type I ulnar nerve compression, Grundberg[42] reported 92% of his patients had a positive Phalen test, but only 44% had a positive Tinel test.[42] If patients have dorsal-ulnar hand paresthesia, a source of compression proximal to the ulnar tunnel should be sought.

Imaging and Electrodiagnostic Studies

Radiographic studies should include the standard posterior-anterior and lateral views in addition to a carpal tunnel view to evaluate for a hook of the hamate fractures. Computed tomography scans

are helpful to identify fractures or other bony abnormalities. MRI can be used to assess for anomalous muscles, ganglion cysts, or ulnar artery abnormalities.[43] **Figs. 4** and **5** show an MRI of a ganglion cyst in the ulnar tunnel. Electrodiagnostic studies can confirm ulnar nerve compression within the ulnar tunnel.[44]

Treatment

Like most compressive neuropathies, initial conservative measures include rest, antiinflammatories, and splinting. Activity modification has proven to be effective when the cause is repetitive trauma or compression.[45] If these measures fail to relieve symptoms, operative release of the volar carpal ligament and exploration of the ulnar nerve and artery are indicated. **Fig. 6** shows the decompression of the deep motor branch of the ulnar nerve after excision of the ganglion cyst shown in **Figs. 4, 5**, and **7**. The palmaris brevis and the antebrachial fascia should be incised to expose the ulnar artery and nerve, which are followed distally to release the fibrous arch of the hypothenar musculature. Surgical outcomes are generally reported as good but because of the rarity and heterogeneity of ulnar tunnel syndrome, there are no comparative studies of interventions or long-term outcomes.[46]

Authors' Experience

In the authors' experience, decompression of the Guyon canal is rarely indicated. Although many

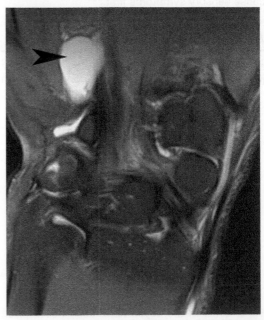

Fig. 4. Coronal section from MRI demonstrating ganglion cyst (*arrowhead*) just distal to the hook of the hamate.

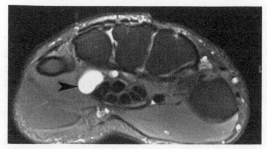

Fig. 5. Axial section from MRI demonstrating ganglion cyst (*arrowhead*) directly ulnar to digital flexor tendons.

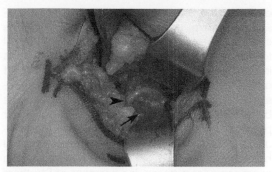

Fig. 7. View from palmar incision demonstrating ganglion cyst (*arrow*) compressing the motor branch of the ulnar nerve (*arrowhead*) against the hook of the hamate (*star*). Leading edge of hypothenar musculature has already been released and contents of carpal tunnel retracted superiorly.

patients presenting with carpal tunnel syndrome will have symptoms throughout all fingers, isolated carpal tunnel release often results in complete symptomatic resolution.[47] This resolution may be secondary to increased volume and decreased pressure within the Guyon canal following the release of the transverse carpal ligament.[41,48–50]

In the authors' practice, they have approached the Guyon canal through either an ulnar-sided approach beginning proximal to the wrist flexion crease and extending into the palm in Bruner-style zigzag fashion or through a carpal tunnel incision just radial to the hook of the hamate. The ulnar-sided approach gives full visualization of the neurovascular bundle, but visualization can be difficult when dissecting through the hypothenar fat pad. Therefore, when using the ulnar-sided approach, the authors strongly recommend the identification of the ulnar nerve and artery in the distal forearm and then dissecting from proximal to distal to expose and decompress the nerve. Alternatively, a carpal tunnel incision can proceed in an ulnar direction superficial to the transverse carpal ligament, which will lead directly

to the Guyon canal. This approach has the advantage of avoiding the hypothenar fat pad (it is kept superficial), and one can visualize the lead edge of the hypothenar musculature at the hook of the hamate to decompress the ulnar nerve. The disadvantage of this incision is the more limited proximal exposure.

When releasing the Guyon canal secondary to extrinsic compression of the ulnar motor branch, the authors have been pleased with their outcomes. Across a wide range of patient ages, excision of ganglion cysts from zone 2 of the Guyon canal has resulted in the return of lost intrinsic motor function within 6 months. When exploring the Guyon canal, the authors have also found an engorged branch of the ulnar artery accompanying the motor nerve branch, which reported symptomatic resolution after decompression of the nerve.

PRONATOR SYNDROME

Pronator syndrome (PS) is the compression of the median nerve proximal to the wrist between the humeral and ulnar heads of the pronator teres muscle. However, the nerve can also be compressed beneath the proximal arch of the flexor digitorum superficialis (FDS); the lacertus fibrosus; the Struthers ligament; or anomalous muscles, such as the Gantzer muscle, an accessory flexor pollicis longus (FPL) muscle.[51–53] PS can be a misleading term because it is often used to describe median nerve compression proximal to the elbow and not just compression at the pronator teres muscle.[2]

Median Nerve Anatomy

The median nerve is formed from the convergence of the terminal divisions of the medial and lateral

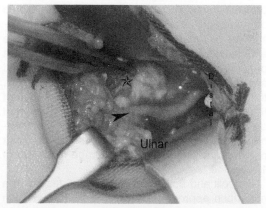

Fig. 6. Same view from palm of the decompressed ulnar motor branch (*arrowhead*) and hook of hamate (*star*) following excision of the ganglion cyst.

cords of the brachial plexus. In the arm, it descends lateral to the brachial artery before crossing anterior to the artery to become medial to the vessel at the level of the coracobrachialis insertion. In the distal third of the arm, the ligament of Struthers is the first site of possible compression of the median nerve. This ligament is a fibrous band that originates on a vestigial supracondylar process, present in approximately 1% of the population, and originates from the anteromedial humeral diaphysis.[2,51,54] In the presence of a supracondylar process, the ligament of Struthers is variably present and inserts onto the medial epicondyle. When present, the median nerve can be compressed as it passes deep to the ligament of Struthers.

The median nerve travels across the elbow medial to the brachial artery, deep to the lacertus fibrosus and volar to the brachialis. It then passes between the 2 heads of the pronator teres muscle: the humeral head, which originates on the medial epicondyle, and the ulnar head, which originates on the coronoid process. The nerve courses deep to the proximal fibrous arch of the FDS and travels between the FDS and flexor digitorum profundus (FDP) muscles in the forearm. In the forearm, the median nerve innervates the pronator teres, flexor carpi radialis, FDS, and palmaris longus muscles. Approximately 5 to 8 cm distal to the lateral epicondyle, the anterior interosseous nerve (AIN) branches from the nerve (typically just distal to the FDS origin) to innervate the pronator quadratus, the FPL, and the FDP to the index and long fingers. Approximately 4.5 cm proximal to the wrist crease, the palmar cutaneous branch originates off the radial side of the median nerve and travels distally between the FCR (flexor carpi radialis) and palmaris longus tendons to provide sensibility in the skin over the thenar eminence and palm.[55] The median nerve continues distally into the carpal tunnel under the transverse carpal ligament, which is the most common site of compression.

Diagnosis

PS typically presents as insidious pain in the volar forearm, grip weakness, and paresthesias to the thumb, index, long, and half of the ring fingers. Generally, the symptoms are dynamic and are exacerbated with repetitive pronation and supination movements. The diagnosis of PS can be challenging because symptoms are similar to carpal tunnel syndrome. However, history and clinical examination can often distinguish between the 2 syndromes. Patients with PS should have a negative Tinel and Phalen sign over the carpal tunnel and

typically do not report nocturnal symptoms because wrist flexion is not involved with the cause.[56] Unlike CTS (carpal tunnel syndrome), patients with PS may describe changes in sensibility over the proximal thenar eminence in addition to finger paresthesia because the palmar cutaneous nerve branch originates distal to the site of compression.

The distinctive physical examination for pronator teres syndrome is tenderness over the PT muscle where the median nerve dives between its 2 heads, approximately 6 cm distal to the elbow crease and 4 cm lateral to medial epicondyle.[57] The tenderness in the forearm is aggravated by resisted forearm pronation and also with resisted long finger PIP joint flexion.[56,58]

Additional Studies

There is controversy about the use of electrodiagnostic studies to diagnose PS. Because it is often a dynamic process, electrodiagnostic studies are often normal.[56,59,60] Workup should include 2 orthogonal radiographs of the elbow to evaluate for a supracondylar process from the anterior humerus, which may indicate compression under the Struthers ligament. Ultrasound can be used to look for extrinsic causes for PS, such as a mass or hematoma, if suspected based on clinical assessment.[61,62]

Management

Like most compressive neuropathies, the first line treatment should include conservative management. For PS, this should include a course of antiinflammatory medication and limiting the aggravating activities. In their review of PS in athletes, McCue and colleagues[58] recommend a 12-week period of conservative management before considering surgical interventions.

Traditionally, a large S incision starting 5 cm proximal to the elbow and extending to the middle of the forearm has been recommended for exposure of all potential sites of compression. The exploration begins at the ligament of Struthers proximally and then the median nerve is followed and decompressed through the lacertus fibrosis, the 2 heads of the pronator teres, and the arch of the FDS (Fig. 8).[58] Hartz and colleagues[56] reported on 36 patients treated operatively with this technique for PS; 78% of their patients had excellent or good outcomes, with an average follow-up of 18 months.

Zancolli and colleagues[57] recently described a mini-open approach that uses a 2.5-cm incision to release the deep fascia of the superficial head of the pronator teres muscle and reported a 93% success rate in patients who were also undergoing

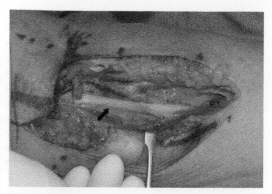

Fig. 8. Anterior approach to median nerve (*arrow*) at elbow with pronator teres (PT) visualized in distal aspect of wound.

carpal tunnel release. In their experience, if the FDS test was negative, only the deep fascia of the superficial head of the PT needed to be decompressed to address pronator teres syndrome.

Lee and colleagues[63] reported the results of performing an endoscopically assisted pronator release in 13 patients diagnosed with PS who had failed an average 5 months of conservative management. All patients had improvement in their postoperative Disability of the Arm, Shoulder, and Hand (DASH) scores; 8 of the 13 had complete resolution of symptoms, whereas 3 had residual arm discomfort.

Authors' Experience

In the authors' practice, PS is diagnosed infrequently. Physical examination and history are first focused on compression at the carpal tunnel. In the setting of intermittent paresthesia in the thumb, index, and long fingers without positive provocative signs over the carpal tunnel, the authors then direct their attention to the cervical spine followed by the proximal forearm. When planning surgery for patients with symptoms of irritability of the median nerve both at the carpal tunnel and proximal forearm, the authors have uniformly treated only the carpal tunnel. In the authors' experience, this has resulted in excellent symptom resolution, and they have not found the need to return to the operating room to address persistent symptoms in the proximal forearm. Therefore, the authors have had rare occasion to decompress the median nerve in the proximal forearm but would not hesitate to do so should conservative measures fail to give relief to patients with provocative findings truly isolated to the proximal forearm.

AIN PALSY

Uncommonly, patients will present with spontaneous loss of active flexion at the thumb interphalangeal and index distal interphalangeal joints. A loss of the index FDP and/or the FPL muscle function has been termed *anterior interosseous nerve syndrome*. This condition may affect each muscle to a variable degree and is not associated with any loss of sensibility.

AIN palsy does not have a clear cause. The condition is most commonly attributed to a postinfectious neuritis or a compression of the AIN after its branching from the median nerve under the leading edge of the FDS origin in the proximal forearm.

AIN palsy has a high rate of spontaneous recovery. Except in the rare case of trauma or mass resulting in nerve dysfunction, surgical decompression of the AIN is not recommended. If there is no return of AIN function (clinical and electrodiagnostic) by 7 to 12 months, then surgical intervention is offered. Operative treatment options include AIN decompression, nerve transfer, or tendon transfer.

Authors' Experience

In the authors' experience, decompression of the AIN has not universally restored function. In cases with recovery of the index FDP but persistent FPL deficit, the authors have found excellent results with the transfer of the brachioradialis or FDS of the ring finger to restore active thumb flexion.

REFERENCES

1. Latinovic R. Incidence of common compressive neuropathies in primary care. J Neurol Neurosurg Psychiatry 2006;77(2):263–5.
2. Dang AC, Rodner CM. Unusual compression neuropathies of the forearm, part II: median nerve. J Hand Surg Am 2009;34(10):1915–20.
3. Carlan D, Pratt J, Patterson JM, et al. The radial nerve in the brachium: an anatomic study in human cadavers. J Hand Surg Am 2007;32(8): 1177–82.
4. Thomas SJ, Yakin DE, Parry BR, et al. The anatomical relationship between the posterior interosseous nerve and the supinator muscle. J Hand Surg Am 2000;25(5):936–41.
5. Abrams RA, Brown RA, Botte MJ. The superficial branch of the radial nerve: an anatomic study with surgical implications. J Hand Surg Am 1992; 17(6):1037–41.
6. Roles NC, Maudsley RH. Radial tunnel syndrome: resistant tennis elbow as a nerve entrapment. J Bone Joint Surg Br 1972;54(3):499–508.
7. Lister GD, Belsole RB, Kleinert HE. The radial tunnel syndrome. J Hand Surg Am 1979;4(1):52–9.
8. Konjengbam M, Elangbam J. Radial nerve in the radial tunnel: anatomic sites of entrapment neuropathy. Clin Anat 2003;17(1):21–5.

9. Verhaar J, Spaans F. Radial tunnel syndrome. An investigation of compression neuropathy as a possible cause. J Bone Joint Surg Am 1991; 73(4):539–44.

10. Kupfer DM, Bronson J, Lee GW, et al. Differential latency testing: a more sensitive test for radial tunnel syndrome. J Hand Surg Am 1998;23(5): 859–64.

11. Hagert CG, Lundborg G, Hansen T. Entrapment of the posterior interosseous nerve. Scand J Plast Reconstr Surg 1977;11(3):205–12.

12. Sarhadi NS, Korday SN, Bainbridge LC. Radial tunnel syndrome: diagnosis and management. J Hand Surg Br 1998;23(5):617–9.

13. Sotereanos DG, Varitimidis SE, Giannakopoulos PN, et al. Results of surgical treatment for radial tunnel syndrome. J Hand Surg Am 1999;24(3):566–70.

14. Moss SH, Switzer HE. Radial tunnel syndrome: a spectrum of clinical presentations. J Hand Surg Am 1983;8(4):414–20.

15. Ritts GD, Wood MB, Linscheid RL. Radial tunnel syndrome. A ten-year surgical experience. Clin Orthop Relat Res 1987;219:201–5.

16. Huisstede B, Miedema HS, van Opstal T, et al. Interventions for treating the radial tunnel syndrome: a systematic review of observational studies. J Hand Surg Am 2008;33(1):72.e1–72.e10.

17. De Smet L, Van Raebroeckx T, Van Ransbeeck H. Radial tunnel release and tennis elbow: disappointing results? Acta Orthop Belg 1999;65(4): 510–3.

18. Lee JT, Azari K, Jones NF. Long term results of radial tunnel release – the effect of co-existing tennis elbow, multiple compression syndromes and workers' compensation. J Plast Reconstr Aesthet Surg 2008;61(9):1095–9.

19. Bolster MA, Bakker XR. Radial tunnel syndrome: emphasis on the superficial branch of the radial nerve. J Hand Surg Eur 2009;34(3):343–7.

20. Lawrence T, Mobbs P, Fortems Y, et al. Radial tunnel syndrome. A retrospective review of 30 decompressions of the radial nerve. J Hand Surg Br 1995; 20(4):454–9.

21. Atroshi I, Johnsson R, Ornstein E. Radial tunnel release. Unpredictable outcome in 37 consecutive cases with a 1-5 year follow-up. Acta Orthop Scand 1995;66(3):255–7.

22. Fitzgerald A, Anderson W, Hooper G. Posterior interosseous nerve palsy due to parosteal lipoma. J Hand Surg Br 2002;27(6):535–7.

23. Werner CO. Radial nerve paralysis and tumor. Clin Orthop Relat Res 1991;268:223–5.

24. Hashizume H, Nishida K, Nanba Y, et al. Non-traumatic paralysis of the posterior interosseous nerve. J Bone Joint Surg Br 1996;78(5):771–6.

25. Vrieling C, Robinson PH, Geertzen J. Posterior interosseous nerve syndrome: literature review and report of 14 cases. Eur J Plast Surg 1998;21(4): 196–202.

26. Dang AC, Rodner CM. Unusual compression neuropathies of the forearm, part I: radial nerve. J Hand Surg Am 2009;34(10):1906–14.

27. Lanzetta M, Foucher G. Entrapment of the superficial branch of the radial nerve (Wartenberg's syndrome). A report of 52 cases. Int Orthop 1993; 17(6):342–5.

28. Calfee RP, Shin SS, Weiss APC. Neurolysis of the distal superficial radial nerve for dysaesthesia due to nerve tethering. J Hand Surg Eur 2008; 33(2):152–4.

29. Dupont C, Cloutier GE, Prevost Y, et al. Ulnar-tunnel syndrome at the wrist. A report of four cases ulnar-nerve compression at the wrist. J Bone Joint Surg Am 1965;47:757–61.

30. Gross MS, Gelberman RH. The anatomy of the distal ulnar tunnel. Clin Orthop Relat Res 1985; 196:238–47.

31. Shea JD, McClain EJ. Ulnar-nerve compression syndromes at and below the wrist. J Bone Joint Surg Am 1969;51(6):1095–103.

32. Jose RM, Bragg T, Srivastava S. Ulnar nerve compression in Guyon's canal in the presence of a tortuous ulnar artery. J Hand Surg Br 2006; 31(2):200–2.

33. Botte MJ, Cohen MS, Lavernia CJ, et al. The dorsal branch of the ulnar nerve: an anatomic study. J Hand Surg Am 1990;15(4):603–7.

34. Ombaba J, Kuo M, Rayan G. Anatomy of the ulnar tunnel and the influence of wrist motion on its morphology. J Hand Surg Am 2010;35(5):760–8.

35. Kuschner SH, Gelberman RH, Jennings C. Ulnar nerve compression at the wrist. J Hand Surg Am 1988;13(4):577–80.

36. Koch H, Haas F, Pierer G. Ulnar nerve compression in Guyon's canal due to a haemangioma of the ulnar artery. J Hand Surg Br 1998;23(2): 242–4.

37. Chen WA, Barnwell JC, Li Y, et al. An ulnar intraneural ganglion arising from the pisotriquetral joint: case report. J Hand Surg Am 2011;36(1):65–7.

38. Patterson JM, Jaggars MM, Boyer MI. Ulnar and median nerve palsy in long-distance cyclists. A prospective study. Am J Sports Med 2003;31(4): 585–9.

39. Akuthota V. The effect of long-distance bicycling on ulnar and median nerves: an electrophysiologic evaluation of cyclist palsy. Am J Sports Med 2005;33(8):1224–30.

40. Murata K, Shih JT, Tsai TM. Causes of ulnar tunnel syndrome: a retrospective study of 31 subjects. J Hand Surg Am 2003;28(4):647–51.

41. Ablove RH, Moy OJ, Peimer CA, et al. Pressure changes in Guyon's canal after carpal tunnel release. J Hand Surg Br 1996;21(5):664–5.

42. Grundberg AB. Ulnar tunnel syndrome. J Hand Surg Br 1984;9(1):72–4.

43. Bordalo-Rodrigues M, Amin P, Rosenberg ZS. MR imaging of common entrapment neuropathies at the wrist. Magn Reson Imaging Clin N Am 2004; 12(2):265–79.

44. Pearce C, Feinberg J, Wolfe SW. Ulnar neuropathy at the wrist. HSS J 2009;5(2):180–3 [quiz: 184–5].

45. Ginanneschi F, Filippou G, Milani P, et al. Ulnar nerve compression neuropathy at Guyon's canal caused by crutch walking: case report with ultrasonographic nerve imaging. Arch Phys Med Rehabil 2009;90(3):522–4.

46. Bachoura A, Jacoby SM. Ulnar tunnel syndrome. Orthop Clin North Am 2012;43(4):467–74.

47. Elfar JC, Calfee RP, Stern PJ. Topographical assessment of symptom resolution following open carpal tunnel release. J Hand Surg Am 2009; 34(7):1188–92.

48. Richman JA, Gelberman RH, Rydevik BL, et al. Carpal tunnel syndrome: morphologic changes after release of the transverse carpal ligament. J Hand Surg Am 1989;14(5):852–7.

49. Ginanneschi F, Filippou G, Reale F, et al. Ultrasonographic and functional changes of the ulnar nerve at Guyon's canal after carpal tunnel release. Clin Neurophysiol 2010;121(2):208–13.

50. Gelberman RH, Hergenroeder PT, Hargens AR, et al. The carpal tunnel syndrome. A study of carpal canal pressures. J Bone Joint Surg Am 1981; 63(3):380–3.

51. Gessini L, Jandolo B, Pietrangeli A. Entrapment neuropathies of the median nerve at and above the elbow. Surg Neurol 1983;19(2):112–6.

52. Horak BT, Kuz JE. An unusual case of pronator syndrome with ipsilateral supracondylar process and abnormal muscle mass. J Hand Surg Am 2008; 33(1):79–82.

53. Bilecenoglu B, Uz A, Karalezli N. Possible anatomic structures causing entrapment neuropathies of the median nerve: an anatomic study. Acta Orthop Belg 2005;71(2):169–76.

54. Campbell WW, Landau ME. Controversial entrapment neuropathies. Neurosurg Clin N Am 2008; 19(4):597–608.

55. Bezerra AJ, Carvalho VC, Nucci A. An anatomical study of the palmar cutaneous branch of the median nerve. Surg Radiol Anat 1986;8(3):183–8.

56. Hartz CR, Linscheid RL, Gramse RR, et al. The pronator teres syndrome: compressive neuropathy of the median nerve. J Bone Joint Surg Am 1981; 63(6):885–90.

57. Zancolli ER III, Zancolli EP IV, Perrotto CJ. New mini-invasive decompression for pronator teres syndrome. J Hand Surg Am 2012;37(8):1706–10.

58. McCue FC, Alexander EJ, Baumgarten TE. Median nerve entrapment at the elbow in athletes. Oper Tech Sports Med 1996;4(1):21–7.

59. Bridgeman C, Naidu S, Kothari MJ. Clinical and electrophysiological presentation of pronator syndrome. Electromyogr Clin Neurophysiol 2007; 47(2):89–92.

60. Rehak DC. Pronator syndrome. Clin Sports Med 2001;20(3):531–40.

61. Jacobson J, Fessell D, Lobo LD, et al. Entrapment neuropathies I: upper limb (carpal tunnel excluded). Semin Musculoskelet Radiol 2010;14(05):473–86.

62. Presciutti S, Rodner CM. Pronator syndrome. J Hand Surg Am 2011;36(5):907–9.

63. Lee AK, Khorsandi M, Nurbhai N, et al. Endoscopically assisted decompression for pronator syndrome. J Hand Surg Am 2012;37(6):1173–9.

64. Younge DH, Moise P. The radial tunnel syndrome. Int Orthop 1994;18:268–70.

65. Jebson PJ, Engber WD. Radial tunnel syndrome: long term results of surgical decompression. J Hand Surg [Am] 1997;22:889–96.

Index

Note: Page numbers of article titles are in **boldface type**.

A

AIN palsy, 451

Alcohol injections, in neuromas, 412

Allografts, nerve, 332–335
    clinical studies for, 334
    for repair of major peripheral nerve injuries, 377–378

Antebrachial cutaneous nerve, neuromas of, 418

Anticonvulsants, in neuromas, 411–412

Antidepressants, tricyclic, in complex regional pain syndrome, 406

Autografts, for repair of major peripheral nerve injuries, 378–379

Axonotmesis, electrodiagnostic changes in, 365

B

Bisphosphonates, in complex regional pain syndrome, 405

Boston Questuionnaire for carpal tunnel syndrome, as outcome measure following rehabilitation of nerve injuries, 388

Bowler's thumb, treatment of, 415, 417

Brachial plexoplasty, 368–369

Brachial plexus, injury of, management of, 393–394

C

Carpal tunnel syndrome, causes and treatment of, 427, 428
    clinical examination in, 429
    clinical outcomes of, 432–433
    clinical presentation of, 427–429
    diagnostic procedures in, 429–430
    differential diagnosis of, 430
    electrodiagnostic studies in, 366–367
        clinic-based, 369
    peripheral nerve injury and, 422–423
    recurrent, **427–434**
    recurrent or persistent, 367
    treatment of, 430–432

CISS, as outcome measure following rehabilitation of nerve injuries, 388

Complex regional pain syndrome, clinical criteria for, 402
    definition of, 402
    epidemiology of, 402–403
    interventions in, 406
    perioperative treatment algorithm for, 404
    prevention of, 402–403
    surgical patients with, 406–407
    treatment of, non-pharmacological, 404
        pharmacologic, 404–406
    with neuropathic pain, treatment algorithm for, 405

Compression neuropathies, uncommon, of upper extremity, **443–453**

Conduits. See *Nerve conduits*.

D

DASH, as outcome measure following rehabilitation of nerve injuries, 387–388

Digital nerve, repair of, immobilization following, 385–386
    recovery based on surgical procedure, 385
    rehabilitation following, 385–386

E

Elbow, ulnar neuropathy at. See *Ulnar neuropathy, at elbow*.
    wrist, and hand, resonstruction of, tendon vesus nerve transfers in, **393–400**

Elbow extension, nerve transfers in, 395

Elbow flexion, nerve transfers in, 395
    tendon transfers in, 395

Electrical stimulation, following repair of major peripheral nerve injuries, 386–387

Electrodiagnostic studies, basics of, 363–364
    timing of, 365–366
        and appropriate use of, **363–369**

Electromyography, needle, 364
    findings after acute neurogenic disorder, 365, 366

Epicondylectomy, medial, in ulnar neuropathy at elbow, 437

F

Fibrin glue, for repair of major periperal nerve injuries, 375–376
    for repair of nerves, 337

Finger extension, merve transfers in, 395–396
    tendon transfers in, 396

Finger flexion, extrinsic, nerve transfers in, 395
    tendon transfers in, 395

Hand Clin 29 (2013) 455–458
http://dx.doi.org/10.1016/S0749-0712(13)00053-X
0749-0712/13/$ – see front matter © 2013 Elsevier Inc. All rights reserved